HOW TO HE
UNTIL THE

First aid can provide a crucial lifeline until professional medical help arrives. You never know when another human being's life — perhaps the life of a loved one or even your own — will depend on your ability to act quickly and intelligently in an emergency. With the ever-increasing pace and complexity of modern living, a sound knowledge of basic first aid is a must for every member of the community.

First aid is never a substitute for medical help. Always send for a doctor as quickly as possible. However, knowing what to do until he arrives can prevent further pain and harm to the victim. You'll find a handy telephone listing for emergency numbers on the inside back cover of this book. Fill in the information **right now.** Seconds can save a life. Keep the book in the same place at all times and be sure every member of your family knows where to find it.

BE PREPARED
BEFORE EMERGENCY STRIKES

Emergencies don't wait, which is why you shouldn't wait until an emergency to study the life-saving steps in this book. It's a good idea to plan several study sessions together with the entire family and, if possible, to get practice in a local first aid class.

This book has been especially designed as a quick-reference for the layman faced with an emergency. It contains step- by-step illustrations and is set in a clear, extra large type for easier reading.

Check for this symbol on any emergency victim who is unable to talk or is in a confused state. It tells you the person needs special care, such as insulin for a diabetic, or that he is allergic to certain drugs, is an epileptic or needs certain medicines. Your doctor can help you get such an identifying card if you need one yourself.

EMERGENCY
FAMILY
FIRST AID GUIDE

A Fireside Book Published by
SIMON AND SCHUSTER

A Fireside Book
Published by Simon and Schuster
A Division of Gulf & Western Corporation
Simon & Schuster Building
Rockefeller Center
1230 Avenue of the Americas
New York, New York 10020

Manufactured in the United States of America

5 6 7 8 9 10 11 12 13 14

ISBN 0-671-21427-6

ACKNOWLEDGMENTS

Sincere appreciation is expressed to the following organizations and individuals for their help in the review and preparation of the material contained in this book:

American Academy of Pediatrics

American Medical Association

Myron I. Buchman — M.D., New York, N.Y.

Norman A. Greene — D.D.S., New York, N.Y.

Frederic Jung — M.D., Chicago, Illinois

Harold Laufman — M.D., Ph.D., New York, N.Y.

Shirley Motter Linde — M.S., New York, N.Y.

Lee Salk — Ph.D., New York, N.Y.

Stuart Scherr — Art Director

Leon J. Taubenhaus — M.D., M. Ph., New York, N.Y.

WHERE TO FIND

(CONTENTS LISTED ALPHABETICALLY)

PAGE

A **ANTIDOTES** (For poisons).... **41-50**

APPENDICITIS **116**

ARTIFICIAL RESPIRATION **1**

    MOUTH-TO-MOUTH RESCUE BREATHING   1
       (Adults/Children/Infants)

    ARM LIFT METHOD 7

    CLOSED-CHEST RESCUE METHOD 9
       (Resuscitation)

    CHOKING 13
    GAS POISONING 12
    DROWNING 15
    ELECTRIC SHOCK 19
    LIGHTNING 23

APOPLEXY (STROKE) **38**

B **BANDAGING** (How to Bandage) **103**

BIRTH (Pregnancy Emergencies) **129**

BITES and STINGS **89**
    ANIMAL BITES 89
    HUMAN BITES 90

EMERGENCY NUMBERS ON INSIDE BACK COVER

WHAT TO DO

(CONTENTS LISTED ALPHABETICALLY)

PAGE

INSECT BITES AND STINGS 91, 95
SNAKE BITE 96

BLACK EYE ... 80

BLEEDING ... 25

STOPPING SERIOUS BLEEDING 25
PRESSURE POINTS 27
TOURNIQUET 29
INTERNAL BLEEDING 32
NOSEBLEED 33
CUTS 77, 80

BLISTERS ... 81
BOILS ... 81
BROKEN BONES ... 69
BRUISES ... 80
BURNS ... 61

SERIOUS BURNS 61
MINOR BURNS 63
CHEMICAL BURNS 64
SUNBURN 65
PREVENTION 65
HEAT ILLNESS 65

EMERGENCY NUMBERS ON INSIDE BACK COVER

WHERE TO FIND

(CONTENTS LISTED ALPHABETICALLY)

		PAGE
C	**CHEST PAINS**	**125**
	CHILDBIRTH	**129**
	CHILLS	**124**
	CHOKING	**13**
	SWALLOWED OBJECTS	132
	CONVULSIONS	**39**
	CUTS	**77,80**
D	**DIARRHEA**	**117**
	DIZZINESS	**37**
	DROWNING	**15**
	ARTIFICIAL RESPIRATION	1
	DRUG EMERGENCY	**117**
	DRUGS	**139**
E	**EARACHE**	**118**
	ELECTRIC SHOCK	**19**
	ARTIFICIAL RESPIRATION	1

EMERGENCY NUMBERS ON INSIDE BACK COVER

WHAT TO DO

(CONTENTS LISTED ALPHABETICALLY)

PAGE

EMOTIONAL PROBLEMS 119
SUICIDE ATTEMPTED 119
VIOLENT BEHAVIOR 120

EYE (Injuries and Problems)..... 122
CHEMICAL BURNS OF EYE 123

F ## FAINTING 40

FAMILY HEALTH (Supplement) 135
HOW TO CHOOSE A FAMILY DOCTOR.. 135
FINDING A DOCTOR IN EMERGENCY... 135
CHECK-UPS 135
IMMUNIZATION 137
IMMUNIZATION SCHEDULE 138
CANCER WARNING SIGNALS 136
DRUGS 139

FEVER 124

FIRST AID SUPPLIES (Basic) 145

FROST 67
FROSTBITE 67
SEVERE COLD 68

EMERGENCY NUMBERS ON INSIDE BACK COVER

WHERE TO FIND

(CONTENTS LISTED ALPHABETICALLY)

PAGE

G **GAS POISONING**
(Carbon Monoxide).............. **12**

GENERAL EMERGENCY **115**

VOMITING 134
NAUSEA 134
STOMACH PAINS 134
APPENDICITIS 116
DIARRHEA 117
DRUG EMERGENCY 117
FEVER AND CHILLS 124
HEMORRHOIDS 127
EARACHE 118
EYE 122
SORE THROAT 132
SWALLOWED OBJECTS 132
HICCOUGHS 128
TOOTHACHE 133
PREGNANCY EMERGENCIES 129
HEART ATTACK 125
EMOTIONAL PROBLEMS 119

GUNSHOT WOUNDS **78**

EMERGENCY NUMBERS ON INSIDE BACK COVER

WHAT TO DO

(CONTENTS LISTED ALPHABETICALLY)

PAGE

H HEAD INJURY (Skull) 71
HEART ATTACK 125
HEAT PROSTRATION (Sunstroke) 66
HEAT EXHAUSTION 66
HICCOUGHS 128

I IMMUNIZATION SCHEDULE 138

L LABOR (Pregnancy Emergencies) 129
LIGHTNING (After it strikes) 23

M MOVING AN INJURED
PERSON 55

N NAUSEA 134
NOSEBLEED 33

EMERGENCY NUMBERS ON INSIDE BACK COVER

WHERE TO FIND

(CONTENTS LISTED ALPHABETICALLY)

PAGE

P POISONS **41**
  SYMPTOMS 45
  INHALED POISONS 46
  ANTIDOTES FOR SPECIFIC POISONS .. 48
  PREVENTION 51
  LEAD POISONING 52
  PLANTS 53
  GAS POISONING (CARBON MONOXIDE) 12

S SHOCK **35**
  SIGNS OF SHOCK 35
  UNCONSCIOUSNESS 37
  ELECTRIC SHOCK 19

SNAKEBITES **96**
SPLINTERS **80**
**SPRAINS/STRAINS/
DISLOCATIONS** **83**
STINGS **91**
STOMACH PAINS **134**
STROKE **38,125**
SUNBURN **65**
SUNSTROKE·Heat Prostration 66

EMERGENCY NUMBERS ON INSIDE BACK COVER

WHAT TO DO

(CONTENTS LISTED ALPHABETICALLY)

		PAGE
	SUPPLIES (First Aid)	145
	SORE THROAT	132
	SWALLOWED OBJECTS	132
T	TEETH CARE	133
	TOOTH PROBLEMS	133
U	UNCONSCIOUSNESS	37
V	VOMITING	134
W	WOUNDS/CUTS/BRUISES	77
	CUTS	77,80
	GUNSHOT WOUNDS	78
	DEEP CHEST WOUNDS	78
	EXPOSED INTESTINES	79
	BRUISES	80
	BLACK EYE	80
	SPLINTERS	80
	BOILS	81
	BLISTERS	81
	FISHHOOKS IN FLESH	81

EMERGENCY NUMBERS ON INSIDE BACK COVER

ARTIFICIAL RESPIRATION

MOUTH-TO-MOUTH METHOD
(or mouth-to-nose)

ADULTS: Blow forcefully, (10-15 breaths per minute) about every 5-6 seconds. Watch victim's chest and stomach for effect.

1. Place victim on his back. Tilt head back so chin points up.

2. Clear the mouth, wipe out mouth with your fingers or handkerchief wrapped around fingers. Remove false teeth.

3. Pull jaw into jutting-out position. Hold mouth open, keeping tongue from falling back into throat with thumb.

1

ARTIFICIAL RESPIRATION

4. Open your mouth wide and "lock" it over victim's mouth so no air escapes. Pinch victim's nostrils shut.

FOR MOUTH-TO-NOSE: Close victim's mouth and "lock" your mouth over victim's nose.

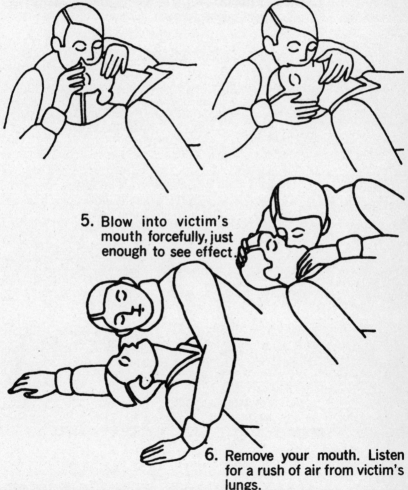

5. Blow into victim's mouth forcefully, just enough to see effect.

6. Remove your mouth. Listen for a rush of air from victim's lungs.

2

ARTIFICIAL RESPIRATION

MOUTH-TO-MOUTH METHOD
(or mouth-to-nose)

SMALL CHILDREN OR INFANTS: *Gently* blow puffs of air at about 20 per minute.

1. Clear mouth with finger, or finger wrapped in handkerchief. Place child on his back. Lift jaw so it juts out as with adults.

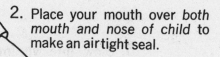

2. Place your mouth over *both mouth and nose of child* to make an airtight seal.

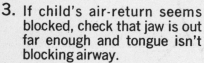
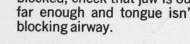

3. If child's air-return seems blocked, check that jaw is out far enough and tongue isn't blocking airway.

ARTIFICIAL RESPIRATION

Begin artificial respiration without delay.
Begin the minute a person's breathing has stopped or if lips, fingernails, or tongue have a blue color to them.

As little as 10 seconds delay can tip the scales between life and death. The average person may die within 3 minutes of the time breathing stops unless you start artificial respiration at once.

The most effective way to help someone who has stopped breathing is to use mouth-to-mouth resuscitation. You blow your breath into the victim's lungs to restart his own breathing system. No help or equipment is necessary. *Even a child can save an adult's life using this method.* You can keep it up for hours without getting tired.

PLACE VICTIM IN FACE UP POSITION AND BEGIN MOUTH-TO-MOUTH STEPS AS SHOWN IN PICTURES

Clear anything in the mouth with your fingers or a handkerchief wrapped around your fingers. If water, mucus, vomit, sand or other material is blocking the air passage, turn victim's head to one side, wipe mouth out, reaching far back into the person's throat, if necessary. If false teeth are present, remove them so they will not block throat.

4

ARTIFICIAL RESPIRATION

HOW TO HANDLE SPECIAL PROBLEMS:

If you don't hear a return rush of air coming from the victim after breathing into his mouth, check to be sure his head is tilted back far enough. Neck skin should be stretched. Check that tongue hasn't fallen back to block air. Correct victim's head position. Begin mouth-to-mouth breathing again.

If you still get no air return from victim:

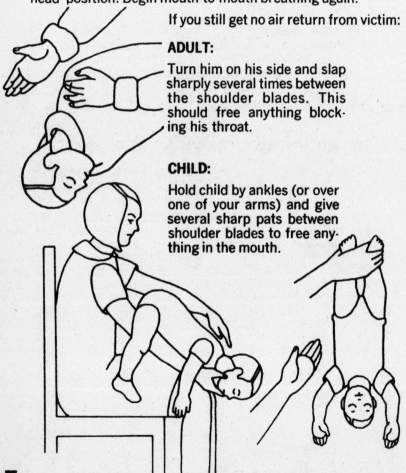

ADULT:

Turn him on his side and slap sharply several times between the shoulder blades. This should free anything blocking his throat.

CHILD:

Hold child by ankles (or over one of your arms) and give several sharp pats between shoulder blades to free anything in the mouth.

5

ARTIFICIAL RESPIRATION

If gurgling or noisy breathing is heard, correct head-back position again. *Be sure nothing is blocking the air passage.*

Do not give up if rescue breathing doesn't work right away. In some cases (like carbon monoxide poisoning and electric shock) rescue breathing must be continued for a very long time. *Continue until the doctor arrives or the person begins breathing for himself.*

If person begins breathing for himself, do not let him sit up or stand for about 30-60 minutes (better still, not until the doctor arrives). Be ready to start mouth-to-mouth breathing again if victim's breathing fades or stops.

BREATHING TUBE AIRWAY OR RESUSCITUBE

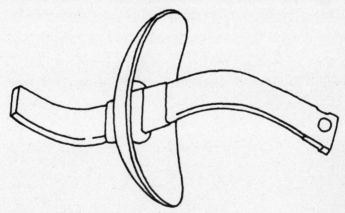

Available at your drugstore. The airway may be used for adults and children over 3 years of age. One end is placed in the mouth of the rescuer, the other end fits over victim's tongue. Using the tube helps avoid direct contact of mouth-to-mouth (or mouth-to-nose) breathing methods. Keep an airway in your home and family car.

6

ARTIFICIAL RESPIRATION

ARM LIFT METHOD:

Always try the mouth-to-mouth rescue method *first*. The Arm Lift Method is far less effective.

Do *not* use if victim has arm injury.

1. Clear victim's mouth with finger or cloth-wrapped finger. Place him face down, one hand on the other. Turn his head to one side so that his chin juts out.

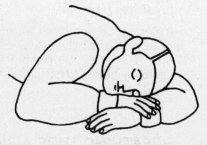

2. *Kneel at victim's head.* Place your hands on flat of his back so your palms rest *in a line* with victim's armpits.

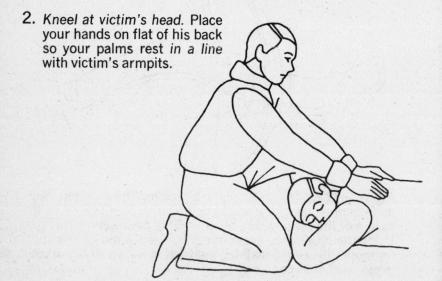

ARTIFICIAL RESPIRATION

3. *Rock forward* until your arms are almost straight up and down. The upper part of your body will be pressing on your hands.

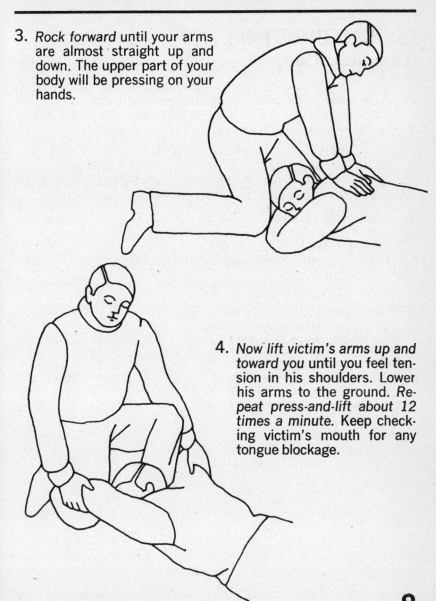

4. *Now lift victim's arms up and toward you* until you feel tension in his shoulders. Lower his arms to the ground. *Repeat press-and-lift about 12 times a minute.* Keep checking victim's mouth for any tongue blockage.

ARTIFICIAL RESPIRATION

CLOSED-CHEST METHOD (FOR ADULTS) (resuscitation)

Use this rescue method only if the victim has already reached a deathlike appearance, stopped breathing, pupils are dilated (look large), and you feel no pulse in the large neck artery just below the ear (about 1½ inches).

This method may damage internal parts if used the wrong way by an untrained first aider. Therefore, use it only when other methods such as mouth-to-mouth breathing fail, or the victim is so close to death that it is your only chance to save him.

1. Place victim on his back on a flat, solid surface. Tilt head back so mouth is open and ready for mouth-to-mouth rescue breathing.

2. Clear mouth with your fingers (or fingers wrapped in a clean handkerchief.) Be sure nothing is blocking the air passage.

3. The exact point to apply pressure is on the *lower* half of the breastbone (sternum). Find it by:

   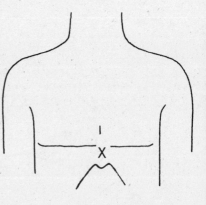

   - Feeling for the soft spot in the lower chest where the breastbone (sternum) ends.
   - The pressure point is one or two fingers above this (see X in picture).

   Pressure must be applied here and nowhere else for this method to work.

ARTIFICIAL RESPIRATION

4.
Kneel at the victim's side. Press down with the *heel of your hand* on the lower breastbone point that you found. Apply a firm heavy pressure. Let your back and body do the work. Press down 1 to 2 inches, once every second.

IF YOU ARE ALONE: **Give** victim *two quick* mouth-to-mouth inflations (see page 1) *for every 15 times* you press down on his breastbone.

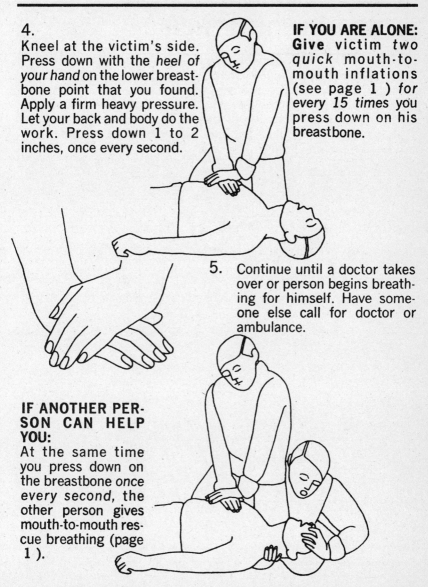

5.　Continue until a doctor takes over or person begins breathing for himself. Have someone else call for doctor or ambulance.

IF ANOTHER PERSON CAN HELP YOU:
At the same time you press down on the breastbone *once every second*, the other person gives mouth-to-mouth rescue breathing (page 1).

10

ARTIFICIAL RESPIRATION

CLOSED-CHEST METHOD
(resuscitation)

FOR SMALL CHILDREN OR INFANTS

- Press with two fingers on the *middle* of the breastbone (sternum). Press down 1 inch 100-120 times a minute (or about twice per second). For older children use the heel of *one* hand only.

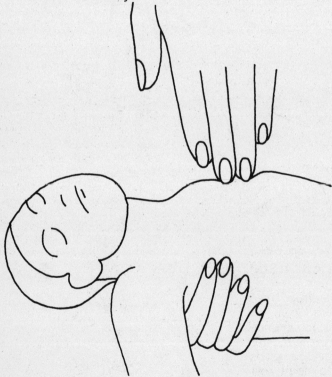

ARTIFICIAL RESPIRATION

GAS POISONING
Carbon Monoxide Poisoning

Get victim into fresh air at once or open all windows. Begin mouth-to-mouth rescue breathing (see page 1) without delay.

You cannot see carbon monoxide, you cannot smell it, but it can take your life without warning. A car engine left running (even for a short time) in a closed garage can cause death. Carbon monoxide poisoning can even occur on the open road if your car has a faulty muffler. Anytime you use a wood or coal fire, a charcoal grill, stove or oil burner in a badly aired room you also risk carbon monoxide poisoning.

SIGNS:

- Headache
- Dizziness
- Weakness
- Skin, lips, nails may be light red
- Difficulty in breathing
- Possibly some vomiting followed by collapse and unconsciousness

Ask Someone to Call for Help

Keep the number of your local poison control center in the back of this book. Do it now, have it ready in case of an emergency. Be sure to tell whomever you call for help to bring oxygen.

12

ARTIFICIAL RESPIRATION

CHOKING: ACT FAST!

Don't even stop to call the doctor, ambulance or police, unless someone can do it for you.

Do not try to grab the object unless you can hook your finger around it. You may push it deeper into the throat. If you can't get it out in 60 seconds take the following actions:

INFANTS AND CHILDREN:

Hold infant by ankles, head straight down. (If bigger child, lay across your arm or leg with head face down.)

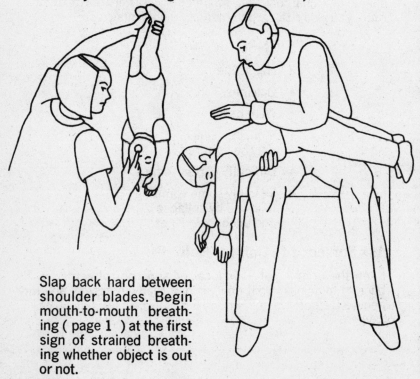

Slap back hard between shoulder blades. Begin mouth-to-mouth breathing (page 1) at the first sign of strained breathing whether object is out or not.

13

ARTIFICIAL RESPIRATION

ADULTS:

Place victim face down over edge of table or bed. Shoulders should hang down.

Slap his back hard between shoulder blades.

Begin mouth-to-mouth breathing if breathing stops or becomes very difficult. Begin even if object is still stuck.

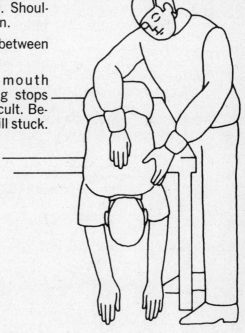

If victim begins struggling for breath, or nails, lips, or tongue are bluish, begin mouth-to-mouth breathing (see page 1) *at once* even if object *hasn't come out*. Blow past it if you must.

PREVENT CHOKING ACCIDENTS:

Keep all small objects out of child's reach. Children like to put things like beans, pits, pins, buttons, coins, beads in their mouth. Never buy a toy smaller than a child's fist. Check toys for parts that could come loose and be swallowed (like a teddy bear's eyes, the wheel on a truck).

14

ARTIFICIAL RESPIRATION

DROWNING

If victim's breathing has stopped, begin mouth-to-mouth rescue breathing (see page 1) as fast as possible, the instant you pull him from the water or even in shallow water (see page 17).

Do not waste your time trying to empty water from his lungs. Swallowed water will not hurt him. But a 10-second delay in beginning mouth-to-mouth breathing could cost his life:

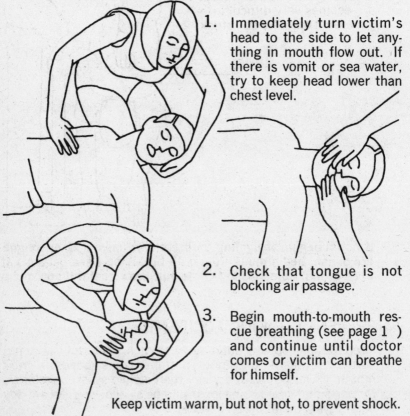

1. Immediately turn victim's head to the side to let anything in mouth flow out. If there is vomit or sea water, try to keep head lower than chest level.

2. Check that tongue is not blocking air passage.

3. Begin mouth-to-mouth rescue breathing (see page 1) and continue until doctor comes or victim can breathe for himself.

Keep victim warm, but not hot, to prevent shock.

ARTIFICIAL RESPIRATION

IN-WATER RESCUE METHODS

(Do *not* attempt in-water rescue unless you are a very good swimmer and familiar with rescue techniques).

DEEP WATER:

Grab hold of victim's head with one hand. Pull head back, mouth should open. Keep holding head back.

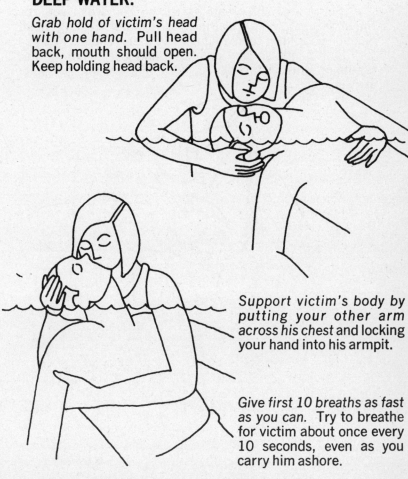

Support victim's body by putting your other arm across his chest and locking your hand into his armpit.

Give *first 10 breaths as fast as you can.* Try to breathe for victim about once every 10 seconds, even as you carry him ashore.

16

ARTIFICIAL RESPIRATION

IN-WATER RESCUE METHODS

NEAR SHORE:

Don't waste time trying to get victim onto dry land when breathing has stopped.

If victim is still not breathing for himself when you reach the shore, stop and kneel in shallow water, resting victim's head on your knee to keep it above water. Hold his head back with both hands so chin points up and give mouth-to-mouth breathing until victim begins breathing for himself or help arrives.

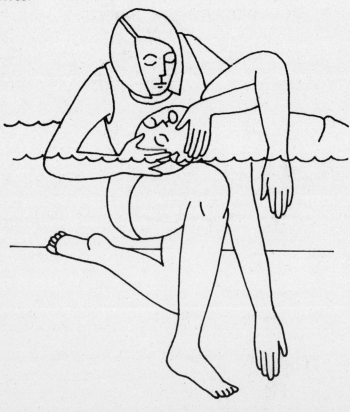

ARTIFICIAL RESPIRATION

When you get victim onto dry land, turn his head to one side. If possible keep his head lower than his chest so vomit and sea water don't go back into his lungs.

Clear the mouth of any mucus, vomit or water with your fingers (or handkerchief-wrapped fingers). Start mouth-to-mouth breathing.

If victim's breathing weakens, or his skin turns bluish, breathe mouth-to-mouth *in beat* with his breathing.

If victim has convulsive attack during rescue, change to the mouth-to-nose method (see page 3).

PREVENT DROWNING ACCIDENTS:

- *Never* leave a small child alone in the bathtub. Not even for a second.

- *Learn to swim,* if possible, well enough to pass the standard Red Cross beginning swimmer's test.

- *Don't take a bath if under sedation* or after you have taken sleeping pills. Adults have drowned in a few inches of water.

ARTIFICIAL RESPIRATION

ELECTRIC SHOCK

Never use anything wet, damp, or metallic when trying to save someone.

Act quickly in cases of electric shock. Electric shock from everyday household current can kill a person or "knock him out." It can *stop* breathing.

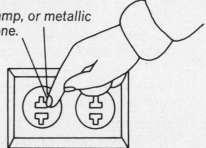

- If someone else is with you, ask him to call the doctor.

- Free victim from the current. *(Danger:* see how on page 21.)

- *Never* touch a victim until he is free of current.

- *If possible, turn off current* (such as light switch). Outdoors: try to get someone to call the electric company to turn off the power. But do not wait for this. Begin rescue. One way is to push victim from current with long board.

- *If breathing has stopped,* begin mouth-to-mouth breathing (see page 1) as soon as it is safe to touch victim directly. Continue until help arrives.

- *Protect yourself.* Put something *dry* under your feet and keep something dry (dry rope, cloth, stick—see page 21) between you and the victim. Wrap hands in dry newspapers or wear *dry* gloves.

- In working near electricity, use one hand rather than two; don't give the current a chance to pass through your heart. Avoid ladders made of metal.

BE CAREFUL: *Do not touch victim* with bare hands until power is turned off or person is no longer touching it. *You may be electrocuted yourself.*

19

REMEMBER
THE EIGHT BASIC LIFE SAVING
STEPS IN FIRST AID
SEE INSIDE FRONT COVER FOR DETAILS

1. Verify breathing. If stopped or very weak, give mouth-to-mouth rescue breathing *at once.*

2. Do not move victim unless absolutely necessary for safety (fire or other danger to life).
   Keep him lying flat on level surface.

3. Stop bleeding. Apply pressure *directly* over wound with a compress or the heel of your hand if that is all you have.

4. Keep injured person warm (but not hot) to prevent shock.

5. Give nothing by mouth if injured person is unconscious or semi-conscious.

6. Calm victim by staying calm yourself.

7. Obtain information for doctor: victim's name, address, nature of injuries.

8. Get medical help fast. Stay with victim. If you can, have someone else telephone for help.

REMEMBER
EMERGENCY NUMBERS ON INSIDE BACK COVER

ARTIFICIAL RESPIRATION

TO FREE VICTIM FROM ELECTRIC CURRENT:

Stand on something dry: dry board, dry rolled newspapers, dry coat (doubled up), dry rubber floor mat from car.

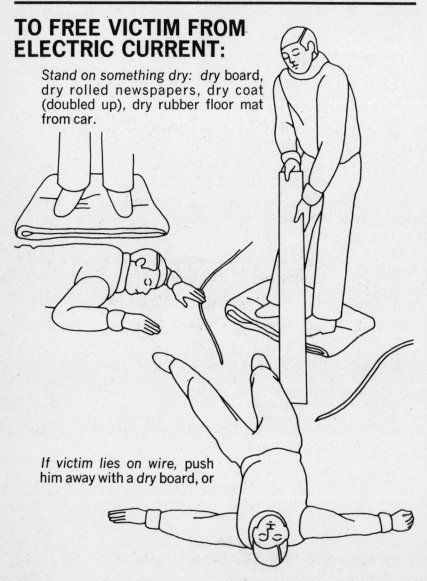

If victim lies on wire, push him away with a *dry* board, or

ARTIFICIAL RESPIRATION

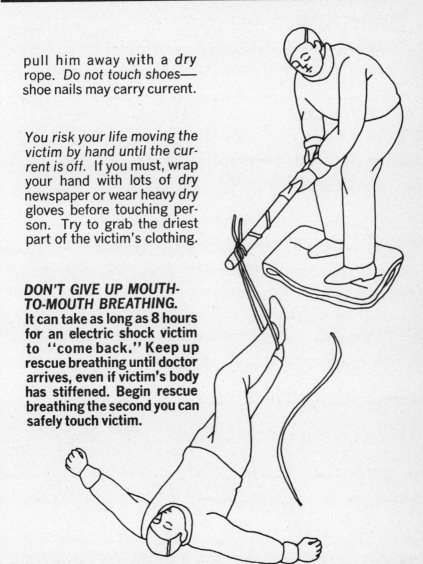

pull him away with a *dry rope. Do not touch shoes*—shoe nails may carry current.

You risk your life moving the victim by hand until the current is off. If you must, wrap your hand with lots of *dry* newspaper or wear heavy *dry* gloves before touching person. Try to grab the driest part of the victim's clothing.

DON'T GIVE UP MOUTH-TO-MOUTH BREATHING. It can take as long as 8 hours for an electric shock victim to "come back." Keep up rescue breathing until doctor arrives, even if victim's body has stiffened. Begin rescue breathing the second you can safely touch victim.

22

ARTIFICIAL RESPIRATION

LIGHTNING

- Victim may be touched right away.
- Begin mouth-to-mouth breathing at once. Continue until doctor arrives.

WHEN LIGHTNING STRIKES

- Keep away from trees that are standing alone.
- You're safe inside a car.
- Run for a ditch, or the lowest hole nearby.

REMEMBER
THE EIGHT BASIC LIFE SAVING
STEPS IN FIRST AID
SEE INSIDE FRONT COVER FOR DETAILS

1. Verify breathing. If stopped or very weak, give mouth-to-mouth rescue breathing *at once.*

2. Do not move victim unless absolutely necessary for safety (fire or other danger to life).
   Keep him lying flat on level surface.

3. Stop bleeding. Apply pressure *directly* over wound with a compress or the heel of your hand if that is all you have.

4. Keep injured person warm (but not hot) to prevent shock.

5. Give nothing by mouth if injured person is unconscious or semi-conscious.

6. Calm victim by staying calm yourself.

7. Obtain information for doctor: victim's name, address, nature of injuries.

8. Get medical help fast. Stay with victim. If you can, have someone else telephone for help.

**REMEMBER
EMERGENCY NUMBERS ON INSIDE BACK COVER**

BLEEDING

BLEEDING

Direct pressure on the wound and elevating the limb will control most bleeding. With heavy bleeding, apply direct pressure as fast as possible.

- *Do not use salves or ointments* on deep wounds.

- *If wound is bleeding profusely,* simply cover with a pressure dressing until medical help becomes available. The loss of blood must be stopped.

- *If you absolutely must clean wound:* clean skin *around* the wound using soap and clean (tap or boiled) water. Scrub your own hands with soap and water first.

- *Always stroke away from wound* when cleaning skin around it.

TO STOP BLEEDING:

1. *Remove all clothing from bleeding area* to see wound clearly. Cut clothing away if necessary. Move victim as little as possible.

2. *Apply direct pressure over the wound* with a sterile dressing, or with a clean folded cloth (shirt, sheet, handkerchief) if no dressing is available.

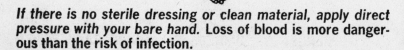

If there is no sterile dressing or clean material, apply direct pressure with your bare hand. Loss of blood is more dangerous than the risk of infection.

25

BLEEDING

3. Keep *steady* pressure over the wound for a few minutes.

4. *If bleeding is in arm or leg, raise the limb above level of body.* Do *not* raise limb if you think there are broken bones.

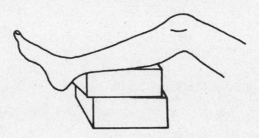

5. *Apply pressure dressing when bleeding stops:* Place gauze compress or folded layers of clean cloth over wound. Never use fluffy absorbent cotton directly on wound. Hold compress with your fingers and bandage into place. *Bandage should not be too tight.* Check. If swelling occurs, loosen the bandage.

If blood comes through the first dressing do not remove it, cover with another layer.

BLEEDING

USE PRESSURE POINTS IF DIRECT PRESSURE ON WOUND DOESN'T STOP BLEEDING

As first steps — always try direct pressure over the wound, a pressure dressing and raising of limb for stopping any serious bleeding. These methods need no special training and can control most bleeding.

Using pressure points closes off blood to the wounded area. Continue direct pressure on the wound even while you hold a pressure point with the other hand.

PRESSURE POINTS:

Bleeding from head, above level of eye: Press against head with finger just in front of ear.

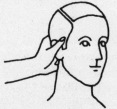

Bleeding below level of eye, above jawbone: Press against hollow spot in jawbone (about an inch in front of angle of the jaw.

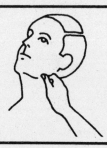

Bleeding from neck, mouth, throat: Hold thumb against back of neck, fingers at side of neck a little below Adam's apple (in hollow just before windpipe, *not over windpipe*). Press finger *toward* thumb.

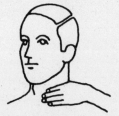

27

BLEEDING

Bleeding armpit, shoulder, upper arm: Fingers or thumb goes in hollow behind victim's collarbone, press against first rib.

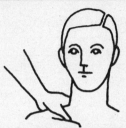

Bleeding from palm: Place thick sterile pad (rolled) in palm, close fingers over it; bandage into closed fist.

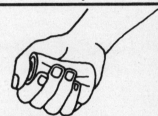

Bleeding from leg: Place heel of hand in middle of depression on inner side of thigh (just below line of groin). Press down against bone.

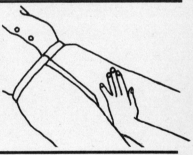

Bleeding below knee: Place pressure pad behind knee, lock lower leg against pad. Tie in place.

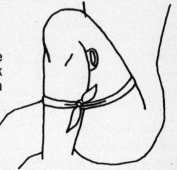

BLEEDING

TOURNIQUET

Whenever you use a tourniquet you risk loss of the victim's limb to save his life. A tourniquet is dangerous and should be used with the *greatest* care. It cuts off blood flow. Gangrene (death of tissues) sets in when blood is stopped for too long.

USE TOURNIQUET *ONLY AFTER* YOU HAVE TRIED EVERY-THING ELSE: Direct pressure, pressure dressing, pressure points, raising limb.

MAKING A TOURNIQUET:

Always keep unbroken skin between wound and the tourniquet.

1. Wrap a wide cloth *twice* around the arm or leg, then tie ends in a *half*-knot. Place a short stick on top.

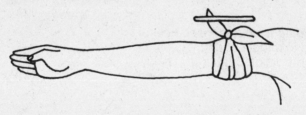

2. *Tie a full* (square) knot over the stick.

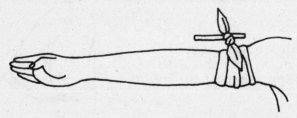

BLEEDING

3. *Twist the stick* to tighten the tourniquet *slightly*. Loosen if the arm or leg turns pale.

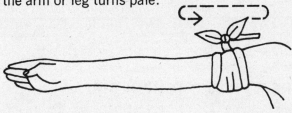

4. *Hold stick in place* with a strip of cloth.

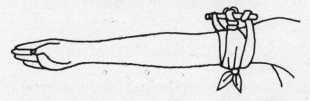

5. *ALWAYS LOOSEN* the tourniquet for a few seconds every 15 minutes until help comes.

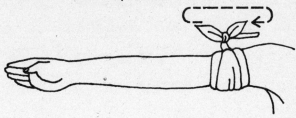

BLEEDING

WHAT TO USE TO MAKE A TOURNIQUET:

In an emergency use any band (about 2 inches wide) long enough to go around arm twice and be tied: belt, stocking, scarf, torn clothing. A good first aid kit should have a tourniquet that buckles. *Do not use wires, ropes, cords* — anything that cuts into flesh.

WHERE TO PLACE TOURNIQUET:

The aim is to get the tourniquet between the injury and the heart. Place it as close to the wound as you can, *but never* on the wound or at the edge of it.

AFTER YOU MAKE THE TOURNIQUET:

*   Get to a doctor *as fast as possible.*

*   If you must leave victim to get help, mark "Tourniquet" or "TK" on his forehead with lipstick, pen, the ashes of a burnt match. *Note time tourniquet was made.*

*   Leave tourniquet in clear view, *do not cover.*

FOR SHOCK

The victim suffers some amount of shock whenever there is serious bleeding.

*   Cover patient, keep comfortable but *not* overheated.

*   Loosen tight clothing.

*   Do *not* give alcohol or any stimulants.

*   Give water only if patient complains of thirst and is able to drink.

31

BLEEDING

INTERNAL BLEEDING

You don't always see signs of internal bleeding. If victim has had a sharp blow or crushing injury to his abdomen, chest or torso, he may well be bleeding inside.

SOME SIGNS OF INTERNAL BLEEDING:

- From stomach—vomit may come out bright red, dark red, black or like large coffee grounds.

- From upper intestines — dark tar-like material in bowel movements.

- From lower intestines — bright red blood in bowel movement.

- From chest and lungs — bright, red, foamy blood coughed up.

Sometimes there are only general signs of internal bleeding: thirst, paleness, weakness, nervousness, anxiety, fast but weak pulse.

IF YOU THINK THERE IS INTERNAL BLEEDING:

- Get a doctor *right away*.

- Keep victim quietly lying down, covered lightly.

- Turn head to one side if there is vomiting or coughing to keep breathing passages clear.

- *If person is having trouble breathing,* the bleeding may be in his lungs. Raise his head a little until he breathes easier.

BLEEDING

NOSEBLEED

Most nosebleeds stop all by themselves. If nosebleeding happens more than once within a short time, see a doctor. Most nosebleeds will stop within 15 to 30 minutes.

BEST WAY TO STOP NOSEBLEED:

- Sit with head bent slightly forward.

- Wet two small pieces of cotton with plain household (3 per cent) peroxide. Squeeze out and insert into lower part of each nostril. (Use cotton alone, if you have no peroxide.)

- Press with your thumb and index finger on either side of *lower* part of nostril, or press over pulse in upper lip.

- Do not talk, eat, drink, or move nose too much.

- Do not change cotton unless you have to.

DO NOT BLOW NOSE, **rub it, sneeze, or pick at dry blood. You may start bleeding again.**

ANOTHER WAY TO STOP NOSEBLEED:

If you don't have peroxide or cotton, hold lower part of nose between thumb and forefinger for 10 to 15 minutes. Breathe through mouth.

Watch out for bleeding into back of throat which can cause clot that may block breathing.

REMEMBER
THE EIGHT BASIC LIFE SAVING
STEPS IN FIRST AID
SEE INSIDE FRONT COVER FOR DETAILS

1. Verify breathing. If stopped or very weak give mouth-to-mouth rescue breathing *at once*.

2. Do not move victim unless absolutely necessary for safety (fire or other danger to life).
   Keep him lying flat on level surface.

3. Stop bleeding. Apply pressure *directly* over wound with a compress or the heel of your hand if that is all you have.

4. Keep injured person warm (but not hot) to prevent shock.

5. Give nothing by mouth if injured person is unconscious or semi-conscious.

6. Calm victim by staying calm yourself.

7. Obtain information for doctor: victim's name, address, nature of injuries.

8. Get medical help fast. Stay with victim. If you can, have someone else telephone for help.

REMEMBER
EMERGENCY NUMBERS ON INSIDE BACK COVER

SHOCK

SHOCK (Unconsciousness, Fainting)

Shock comes with most serious injuries or burns. Treat it at once to help save lives:

- *Send for a doctor.*
- *Take emergency steps called for by the injury. Stop severe bleeding (see page 25); start mouth-to-mouth breathing if needed (see page 1).*
- *Treat for shock even if no signs have appeared yet.*

SIGNS OF IMPENDING SHOCK:

Patient feels weak, and restless.

Pulse is fast but weak.

Face is pale.

Skin feels cold and damp to touch; forehead and palms are sweaty.

Chills.

Nausea.

Breathing not regular or deep.

A person already in shock is silent, limp and motionless. His breathing is inadequate, his pulse weak, and his pupils dilated.

If several of these signs appear, even without known injury, call a doctor.

SHOCK

FIRST AID FOR SHOCK

1. Have patient lie flat on back. Keep him calm and quiet.

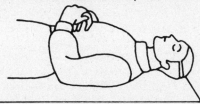

2. Cover him lightly. Protect from cold or wet ground. *Do not* make victim *too* warm. Just keep him from losing too much body heat.

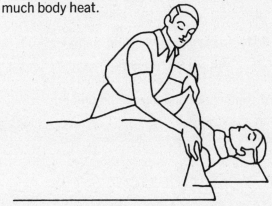

3. Lower victim's head or raise feet slightly to help blood get to heart and brain UNLESS there are injuries to head or legs.

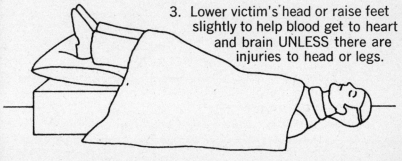

DIZZINESS

Dizziness is not usually serious unless persistent. Have the dizzy person lie down quietly in a comfortable position with eyes closed.

If the room seems to spin around and there is nausea or vomiting, call a doctor.

See a doctor if *any* dizziness lasts a long time or keeps coming back.

UNCONSCIOUSNESS

Unconsciousness is a sign of some illness or injury. *If you know the cause*, such as poisoning, drowning, sunstroke, choking, *give first aid for the cause.* (Look it up in this book.)

Call a doctor if the person does not come around quickly. If there was *any blow to the head*, call a doctor anyway.

Never give an unconscious person anything to drink.

If the victim is a stranger, see if he is carrying *an identification card or tag that says he has diabetes or other illness.* It will have instructions on it.

HOW TO TREAT UNCONSCIOUSNESS

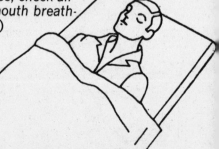

- *If breathing is poor or stops, check airway and start mouth-to-mouth breathing at once.* (See page 1 .)

- Put patient flat on back, keep warm but not hot, loosen tight clothes.

- Look for cause, give proper first aid, call for help if needed.

APOPLEXY (STROKE)

APOPLEXY (STROKE)

Call a doctor at once. This is a very serious cause of uncon-sciousness. It is caused by blood leaking into the brain from a broken blood vessel or a clot which stops blood from reaching part of the brain. Stroke is more likely in an older person, but can also occur in young or middle-aged persons.

SIGNS OF STROKE

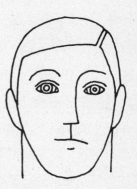

- Face is red or pale grey.
- Pupil of one eye is usually but not always larger.
- Part of body is weak or cannot be moved voluntarily by the person.
- One corner of mouth droops.
- Difficulty in speaking.
- Unconsciousness.

WHAT TO DO IF
PATIENT SHOWS SIGNS OF STROKE

- *Call doctor right away.*
- Keep patient quiet, fairly warm.
- Put cold cloth on head.
- If breathing is difficult or stops, begin mouth-to-mouth breathing. (See page 1 .)

38

CONVULSIONS (Fits)

CONVULSIONS

In a convulsion, *the body gets stiff and moves jerkily.* The person *cannot control his movements* and is usually *unconscious.*

Convulsions can come from a very high fever or other causes. *The danger is that the person may hurt himself.* Take these steps to protect the patient:

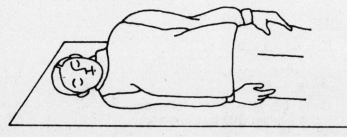

Loosen tight clothing. Take away hard or sharp objects that could hurt the patient.

Call a doctor if convulsion lasts more than 15 minutes or if the patient stays unconscious. Tell your doctor about a convulsion even if it ends quickly.

FANTING

FAINTING

In a fainting spell, the victim is very pale. If a person faints or feels faint, get more blood to flow to the brain:

Lying down helps a person who feels he is going to faint.

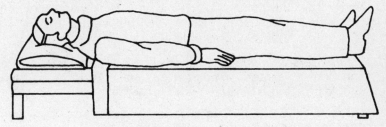

Sitting with head down helps, too.

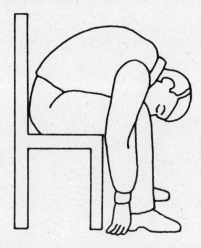

If faint feeling lasts or if fainting happens often, see a doctor.

POISONS

POISONS

Even before you phone for the doctor, cut power of poison *at once* by:

1. Having person spit and vomit if possible, (see list, page 43).

2. Diluting the poison by having him drink water or other "safe liquids" (see below). Do this before looking up specific antidotes. Speed is vital.

If third person is with you, ask them to phone the doctor, Poison Control Center, or nearest hospital. All three numbers should be listed in the back of this book right now.

DO NOT GIVE LIQUIDS to any victim who is semi-conscious, unconscious (not awake), or convulsive.

"SAFE LIQUIDS":

Tap water, milk or raw egg-white in water.

41

POISONS

Fluids may cause vomiting. This is, in many instances, good. Prevent vomitus from entering lungs and causing further damage:

- *Put child* across lap with head down

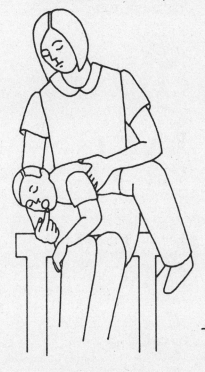

- Adults must lie on stomach with head lower than hips. If head cannot hang over edge of bed, turn head to one side.

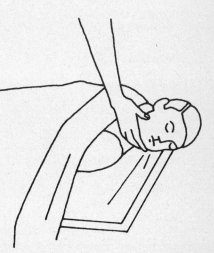

POISONS

DO	DO NOT
MAKE PERSON VOMIT FOR ANYTHING LISTED BELOW; CALL DOCTOR	**MAKE PERSON VOMIT IF ANYTHING ON THIS LIST WAS TAKEN; CALL DOCTOR**

DO	DO NOT
(Except if person is unconscious or half-conscious)	Ammonia
	Benzine
	Bleach (Household)
After-Shave Lotions	Carbolic Acid Disinfectants
Alcohol (Rubbing, Ethyl)	Corn and Wart Removers
Alcohol (Wood, Methyl)	Creosote
Ant and Mouse Baits	Detergents
Antifreeze	Drain Cleaners
Antiseptic Detergents	Dry Cleaning Fluids
Arsenic Rat Poison	Floor Wax and Polishes
Borax	Furniture Wax and Polishes
Camphor and Moth Repellents	Gasoline
Canned Heat	Grease Removers
DDT Insect Poisons	Gun Cleaners
Deodorants	Hair Straighteners
Dry Shampoos	Ink Eradicators
Fireworks	Kerosene
Flea Powder	Lighter Fluid
Formaldehyde	Lime
Freckle Remover	Lye
Hair Dyes	Lysol
Ink	Metal Cleaners
Liniments	Naphtha
Liquor or Beer in Large Amounts	Oven Cleaners
Matches	Paint Brush Cleaners
Nail Polish	Paint Thinners and Removers
Nail Polish Removers (Acetone)	Pine Oil
	Plastic Cement
	Rubber Cement
	Rust Removers

43

POISONS

DO	DO NOT
MAKE PERSON VOMIT FOR ANYTHING LISTED BELOW; CALL DOCTOR	**MAKE PERSON VOMIT IF ANYTHING ON THIS LIST WAS TAKEN; CALL DOCTOR**
Paints	Sodium Carbonate
Perfume	Strong Acids
Permanent Wave Solution (Neutralizers)	Strychnine Rat Poisons
Shellac	Toilet Bowl Cleaners
Shoe Polishes	Turpentine
Silver Polish	Typewriter Cleaners
Sun Tan Preparations	Varnish Removers
Varnishes	Washing Soda
	Wood Preservatives
Always give "safe" fluids or universal antidote before doing anything else.	*Many household mixes have lye in them.* This may rupture the person's esophagus if vomited. Also, petroleum products, such as kerosene, may pass into lungs and damage them if vomited.

HOW TO MAKE PERSON VOMIT

- Place finger or the handle of a spoon at the back of the throat.
- Give warm soap solution or two tablespoons of table salt in a glass of warm water.
- May give one ounce Syrup of Ipecac.
- Keep giving fluids until vomited liquid is clear.

DO NOT MAKE A PERSON VOMIT IF:

- **Already vomiting**
- **Mouth or throat burns**
- **Person is unconscious, semi-conscious, or having convulsions (fits)**

44

POISONS

If Patient is Semi-Conscious, Unconscious, Shows Signs of Shock or Has Difficulty Breathing

- If breathing stops, give mouth-to-mouth rescue breathing at once. (See page 1.)

- Keep mouth clear, keep patient covered, warm.

- Rest patient on stomach, head low and turned to one side.

- Wipe secretions from mouth with handkerchief or finger.

- Extend neck and tilt head upward to keep tongue from falling back and blocking air passage.

- Always try to save container poison came in; if medicine, save all that is left in bottle, bring it to doctor or hospital.

COMMON SYMPTOMS OF POISONING

Always call a doctor if poisoning is suspected. Don't wait for symptoms to develop, but give immediately "safe" fluids or "general antidote."

Call doctor if any of these symptoms occur: nausea and vomiting; cramps; diarrhea; chills or fever; burning of mouth or throat; excessive drowsiness or difficulty in being awakened.

Appendicitis and other illnesses can cause similar symptoms.

Suspect food poisoning if more than one person in the family becomes ill after eating the same foods. Illness from food poisoning may show up in a few minutes or not until a day or two after eating bad food.

45

POISONS

INHALED POISONS

This is probably the most dangerous of all because the victim doesn't know he is in danger. Use the following substances only in rooms that are airy and try not to breathe any vapor for too long a time:

USE ONLY IN WELL-AIRED ROOM

Alcohol (Wood, Methyl)
Ammonia
Antifreeze
Benzene
Carbon Monoxide
Carbon Tetrachloride and other dry-cleaning fluids
Demothing Agents (Naphthalene)
Fire Extinguishing Fluids
Flea Powder
Formaldehyde
Fumigants (Cyanide)
Nail Polish Removers (Acetone)
Paint Removers
Paints
Rat Poisons (Phosphorus, Arsenic)
Shellacs
Stove and Shoe Polishes
Turpentine
Varnishes
Burning of Lead Storage Battery Casings

Bleach and powerful household cleaners for toilet bowls or ovens *should NOT* be mixed with ammonia or vinegar. Such combinations can give off chlorine gas or other harmful gases.

POISONS

WHAT TO DO WITH INHALATION VICTIM

- Carry or drag the victim (do not let him walk) to fresh air immediately.

- Open all doors and windows.

- Loosen all tight clothing.

- If breathing has stopped or is uneven, begin mouth-to-mouth breathing (see page 1).

- Call doctor.

- Keep the person warm. Wrap him in blankets and keep him as quiet as possible.

- If he is having convulsions, keep him in bed in a semidark room and avoid jarring or noise.

- DO NOT GIVE ALCOHOL IN ANY FORM.

- Protect yourself from becoming victim to the poison.

After You Take Emergency Steps

Put patient to bed to keep him warm. After nausea and vomiting stop, give a lot of lukewarm water, fluids. If there is no diarrhea, give salt water enema: 1 teaspoon of salt to a quart of water. Or give a big dose of Epsom salts by mouth.

Save whatever substance caused poisoning for analysis. If you don't know what caused poisoning, save sample of patient's vomitus for analysis. In case of drug overdose, get prescription number, phone and name of pharmacist so poison can be identified quickly.

POISONS

ANTIDOTES FOR SPECIFIC POISONS

If poison is known and you've already given the general first aid treatment (which may or may *not* include forcing patient to vomit), you can take these additional steps if medical help has not yet arrived:

ALKALIS, CAUSTIC

Lye
Ammonia
Drainpipe cleaners
Quicklime
Washing soda

Do not force vomiting. Give acid fruit juices, such as juice of 4 lemons in pint of water.

Or, slightly diluted vinegar. Follow with two or three raw egg whites in water.

Or, salad oil, cooking oil, melted butter.

Or, glass or two of milk.

ACIDS, STRONG

Battery acid
Sulfuric
Nitric
Hydrochloric

Do not force vomiting. Give a teacupful of milk of magnesia.

Or, 2 tablespoons of baking soda in pint of water. Then, raw egg whites in water.

Or, glass or two of milk.

Or, salad oil, any vegetable oil, about ¼ glass.

ANTIDOTES CONTINUED OVER

48

POISONS

ANTIDOTES (Continued)

PETROLEUM DISTILLATES

Kerosene
Gasoline
Benzine
Naphtha
Lighter fluid
Inflammable
  cleaning fluids

Do not force vomiting (danger of aspiration pneumonia).

Give ½ cup of mineral oil.

Give stimulant: strong coffee, tea.

Keep warm, combat shock.

Give artificial respiration if necessary.

"SLEEP DRUG" OVERDOSE

Barbiturates
Sedatives
Opiates
Codeine
Morphine
Paregoric

If conscious, give emetic to induce vomiting.

Give strong black coffee.

Keep patient awake — slap face with wet towel, walk him about, but do not exhaust him.

Give artificial respiration if necessary.

SALICYLATE DRUG OVERDOSE

Aspirin
Headache and cold
  pills
Oil of wintergreen

Induce vomiting unless it has occurred.

Give Syrup of Ipecac.

Or, weak baking soda solution
  (1 teaspoon to pint).

Give strong coffee.

POISONS

CARBOLIC ACID

Phenol (ingredient
    of common
    disinfectants)
    often called
    carbolic acid
Creosote
Creosol disinfectants

Give soapsuds immediately.

Or, give Epsom salts (2 tablespoons to pint of water).

Then, large amounts lukewarm water. (Do Not give any strong emetic).

Also, give thin "soup" of flour or cornstarch in water.

Or, raw egg whites in water.

Do Not give alcoholic drinks.

IODINE

Give flour or cornstarch in water; bread; large amounts of starchy substances.

Follow with emetic to induce vomiting.

Repeat starch and emetic until vomited material has no blue color.

WOOD ALCOHOL

Rubbing alcohol
Denatured alcohol
Methanol

Induce vomiting. (Page 44.)

Give tablespoon of baking soda in quart of warm water.

Repeat emetic and soda solution.

Follow with glass of milk containing teaspoon of baking soda.

50

POISONS

HOW TO PREVENT TRAGEDIES

- Keep prescriptions, household cleaners, insecticides, gasoline, turpentine, kerosene and such out of the reach of children. A locked cabinet is best.

- Never put non-foods in containers used for food.

- Never put anything on food shelves *but* food.

- Never tell children pills taste like candy.

- Never take medicine without reading labels.

- If label is missing, throw medicine bottle away.

- Teach children not to eat strange berries, plants or fruits.

- Protect skin when using solvents and strong cleaning agents as some chemicals can be absorbed through the skin.

- Wash insecticides from skin *immediately* with soap and water.

- Do *not* use outdoor paint which contains lead on anything in your house, especially if children live in your home.

- Write the number of your doctor, hospital nearest you and your nearest Poison Control Center in the space on the inside back cover of this book.

- Instruct baby sitters on emergency measures. Leave this book near the phone for your sitter.

POISONS

LEAD POISONING

Lead poisoning can be fatal or result in paralysis, permanent brain damage or mental retardation. *It occurs mainly in small children who eat pieces of dried paint from walls* or peelings which drop from ceilings. They may chew on window putty, a little at a time.

Never use outdoor paint which contains lead on any indoor furniture or wall. Get in touch with a doctor if any of these symptoms appear. They are noticed gradually.

- Poor appetite
- Stomachache
- Repeated vomiting
- Constipation
- Headaches
- Paleness
- Crankiness
- Convulsions
- Coma

POISONS

POISON IVY, POISON OAK, OR POISON SUMAC

DON'T SCRATCH. This spreads the irritant poison and can cause infection.

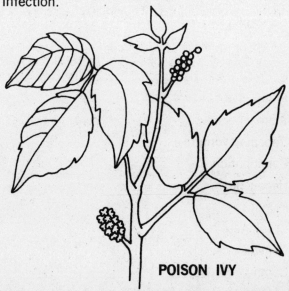

POISON IVY

- You may avoid or minimize rash if you wash all exposed skin thoroughly as soon as possible after exposure to get irritating poison off the skin. Aromatic spirits of ammonia is best; soap and water will do.

- Wash contaminated clothing and let it hang in the air several days before wearing it again.

- Use calamine lotion or cold compresses to help soreness and reduce itching.

- Starch baths are soothing.

- Don't use aerosol first aid sprays. They sometimes make the skin sensitive and the condition worse.

53

POISONS

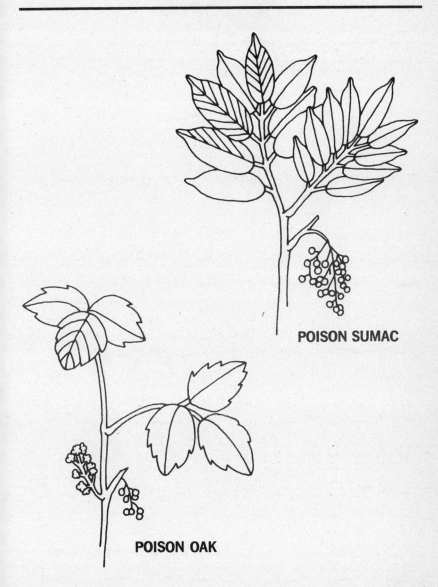

POISON SUMAC

POISON OAK

MOVING AN INJURED PERSON

MOVING AN INJURED PERSON

Never move an injured person unless you have to for his own safety (to get him away from traffic, fire, or other major danger). Always *try* to wait for medical help to arrive. An untrained person can cause serious problems by moving a hurt person incorrectly.

MOVING A VICTIM BY YOURSELF

(If no help is available and you must move victim).

IF VICTIM CAN WALK:

One arm supports victim around his waist. The other holds the victim's arm *nearest* you around your neck.

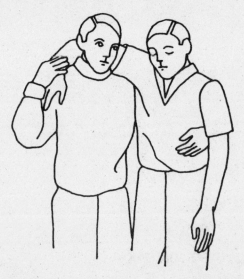

55

MOVING AN INJURED PERSON

NORMAL CARRYING POSITION:

Lean slightly when carrying person.

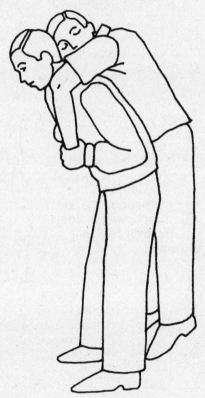

MOVING AN INJURED PERSON

FIREMAN'S CARRY:

1. When person is too heavy to be carried normally, place him face down and kneel at his head facing him:

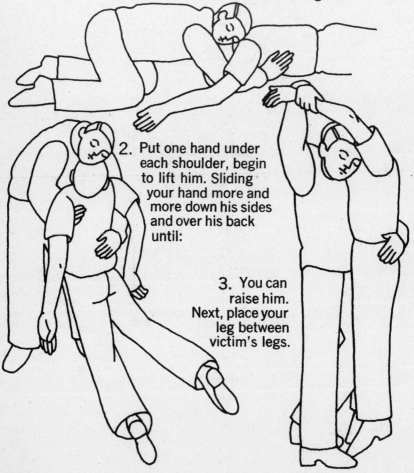

2. Put one hand under each shoulder, begin to lift him. Sliding your hand more and more down his sides and over his back until:

3. You can raise him. Next, place your leg between victim's legs.

MOVING AN INJURED PERSON

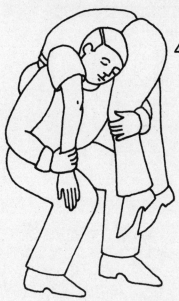

4. Take hold of victim's left lower thigh with your left hand, balance victim across your shoulder, raise yourself up and walk.

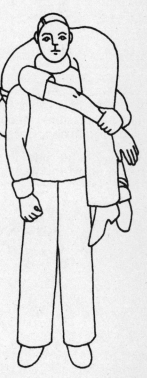

5. Take his left wrist with your right hand. Slip your head under his left arm, lifting his arm around the back of your neck.

If you need to free your right hand later, take hold of victim's left hand in your left hand.

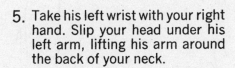

58

MOVING AN INJURED PERSON

MOVING A PERSON WHO IS UNCONSCIOUS
and too heavy to carry in your arms:

1. Lie down even with victim, place your back to his chest. Reach back and bring his upper arm *over* your shoulder and hold it in place with your hand.

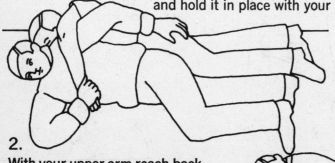

2.

With your upper arm reach back and take hold of victim's clothing (at his hip). Keep holding and roll him on top of your back.

Get up onto one knee, then stand up all the way.

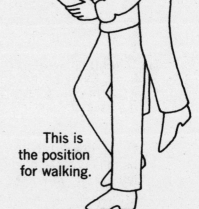

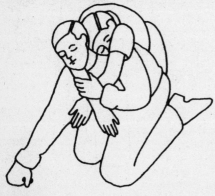

This is the position for walking.

MOVING AN INJURED PERSON

MOVING VICTIM WITH THE HELP OF OTHERS

(It takes two to four people to move an injured adult properly.)

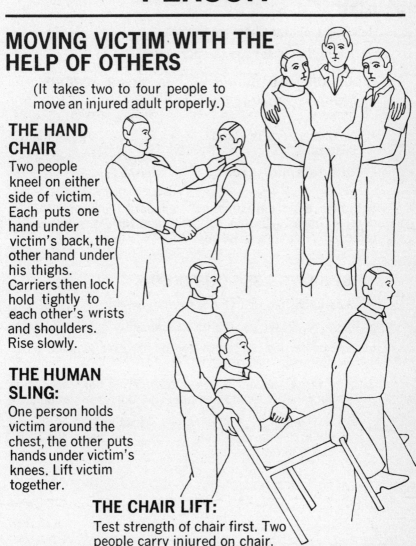

THE HAND CHAIR

Two people kneel on either side of victim. Each puts one hand under victim's back, the other hand under his thighs. Carriers then lock hold tightly to each other's wrists and shoulders. Rise slowly.

THE HUMAN SLING:

One person holds victim around the chest, the other puts hands under victim's knees. Lift victim together.

THE CHAIR LIFT:

Test strength of chair first. Two people carry injured on chair.

For flat carrying position, see page 98.

BURNS

BURNS

(See page 64 for Chemical Burns.)

Decide first how serious the burns are:

MINOR OR MILD BURNS

- Skin is red, *but not broken.*

- No blisters or a few small blisters.

- Only a *small area is burned.*

See page 63 for treatment of minor burns. A burn is *not* minor if it covers a large area.

MAJOR OR SERIOUS BURNS

- *Skin is broken.*

- *Blisters, large or many.*

- *More than a small area is burned.*

If ANY ONE of these signs appears, the burn is serious. Follow the steps below.

FIRST AID FOR SERIOUS BURNS

- *When possible, get victim to the hospital AT ONCE.*

- *If you CANNOT get victim to a hospital take these steps:*

  1. *Put burned part (arm, leg or hand) in ice cold water.* Use basin, pail or bowl.

  2. *If large areas of body are burned,* do not treat patient yourself. Get help at once. Call doctor or ambulance.

  3. *To help stop pain*—cover the patient with a blanket, sheet or even a piece of clothing. This keeps the air out and relieves pain.

BURNS

FIGHT SHOCK

If the patient is thirsty, shock may be starting.

Shock, caused by loss of fluid from the body, is a serious danger with bad burns.

If the patient is conscious (awake) and is NOT vomiting, give him liquids to drink. Give water with salt (1 teaspoon/quart), *but do not give liquids if unconscious or vomiting.*

Give liquids *slowly,* about one cup every hour.

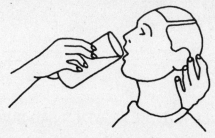

WHAT NOT TO DO FOR SERIOUS BURNS

- **Do NOT pull clothing from bad burns. Leave alone.**

- **Do NOT put ointments, grease or antiseptics on bad burns.**

- **Do NOT open blisters.**

- **Do NOT treat yourself if medical help is near.**

BURNS

TREATING MINOR BURNS

You can't always tell which is a minor burn as the signs of a burn may be delayed for as long as twelve hours. What appears as a minor burn may end up being a major burn. Call a doctor. Don't take chances!

A burn is NOT minor if it covers a large area.

1. Hold the burned part under cold running water *or* hold it in a bowl of *clean* ice cold water for several minutes.

2. Wash with soap and water.

3. For painful minor burns, cover with:

   • A paste made from baking soda mixed with a little water.

   • *Or* a burn ointment.

   NEVER PUT THE ABOVE ON BAD BURNS.

4. Cover the burn with a sterile bandage.

The best way to help the pain is to keep air out by covering the burn.

WHAT TO DO IF CLOTHES CATCH FIRE:

• **If you are alone when your clothes catch fire, *lie down and roll over slowly on the floor until the flames are out.***

• **If another person's clothes are on fire, have him lie down while you *use a rug, a blanket or a heavy coat to put out the flames.***

63

BURNS

CHEMICAL BURNS

Treat at once and call a doctor.

Strong liquids like acids or lye cause very serious burns.

Put victim under the bathroom shower right away. Turn cold water on full. Take off victim's clothing. Run water until all of the chemical is washed away.

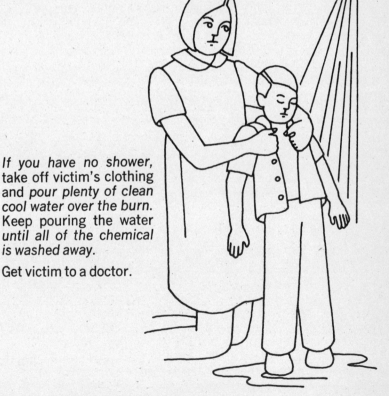

If you have no shower, take off victim's clothing and pour plenty of clean cool water over the burn. Keep pouring the water until all of the chemical is washed away.

Get victim to a doctor.

Chemical burns of eye, see page 123.

BURNS

SUNBURN

For bad sunburn or if there are many blisters (intact or broken), if the person has chills or nausea, or if he vomits, or if the burn covers a large area, or is very painful, *call a doctor.*

For Mild Sunburn

Use any bland, soothing lotion or cream. If none is on hand, a cold cream or cooking oil or salad oil may ease the pain.

PREVENTING SUNBURN

Preventing sunburn: **On your first day in the sun, *do NOT stay uncovered in the sun for long.* If you have very light skin, 5 minutes may be enough. *Half an hour is the most for anyone.***

PREVENTING BURNS

Small children are in most danger from burns.
Prevent trouble:

- *Keep handles of pots and pans away from the edge of the stove so children cannot reach them.*

- *Do NOT leave hot liquids on a table with a cloth on it.* A child can pull on the cloth and spill the liquid on himself.

- *Do NOT leave a child alone in the bathtub.* He may turn on the hot water and be badly burned.

- *Keep children away from matches, stoves, heaters, radiators, open fires, hot food and liquids.*

HEAT ILLNESS

Any person who has been too long in extreme heat or a hot sun may become ill. Working in heat, sweating a great deal and drinking water may cause illness. Sunstroke or Heat Prostration can cause death.

BURNS

SIGNS OF IMPENDING SUNSTROKE
(Heat Prostration)

Most serious. Call a doctor.

- Skin is very hot and dry.
- Mouth temperature is 100 degrees or more.
- Person feels weak, dizzy nauseated and confused.
- Person may not be able to move, may be irrational or unconscious.

TREATMENT

Act quickly. Victim could die.

- Call your doctor.
- Get victim into cool place.
- Have him sit or lie down quietly.
- Wrap body in sheet wet with cold water.

Fan to promote evaporation and help bring down body heat.

Rub patient's arms and legs to carry cooled blood from skin to inside of body.

If patient is unconscious, take him to a hospital.

SIGNS OF HEAT EXHAUSTION
Less serious, but needs treatment.

- Person may get heat cramps after long, hard work in a hot temperature. (Large muscles of legs, shoulders, and arms may contract in painful spasms.)

TREATMENT
- Put patient in a cool airy place.
- Have him sit or lie down quietly.
- Loosen clothing.
- Give sips of water with a little salt in it (use one teaspoon of salt for one pint of water.) Do not give large amounts of water without also giving salt.

If patient still feels ill after several hours, call a doctor.

66

FROST

INJURY FROM COLD OR FREEZING

FROSTBITE

Frozen parts look white or gray and are numb (have no feeling). In frostbite, parts of the body are frozen (usually hands, feet, face or ears). There is no pain in frozen parts.

Call a doctor at once for bad cases of frostbite.

Even in mild cases, check with a doctor later.

WHAT TO DO:

- Thaw frozen parts carefully. *Do NOT rub.*
- *Outdoors, warm the frozen part against the body.* Put hands under armpits or between thighs. Warm ears or nose with the hands.
- *Indoors, put the frozen part in warm, NOT hot, water.* Or cover the frozen part with warm towels or blankets.
- Do not give whiskey or other alcoholic drinks.

WHAT NOT TO DO:

- *NEVER rub with snow or anything else. Frozen areas are easily hurt.* You can cause permanent damage by rubbing.
- *Never use strong heat, such as stove, radiator, hot water or heat lamp, electric blanket or heating pad.*

FROST

LONG EXPOSURE TO SEVERE COLD
A person out in very cold weather for a long time may show these signs:

- Whole body is chilled, may even be numb.
- Person becomes sleepy, may faint.

IF THE VICTIM APPEARS VERY DROWSY:

- Call a doctor.
- Get patient to a warm place.
- Put him in a bathtub full of warm water.
- Then wrap in warm blankets and put him to bed.
- Give warm drinks.
- *If breathing is very poor or stops, begin mouth-to-mouth breathing (* see page 1 *).*

BROKEN BONES

BROKEN BONES

A simple fracture: If the skin is *unbroken;* the fracture is called simple, no matter how many pieces there are because there is little danger of infection.

A compound fracture: If the skin is *broken,* the fracture is called compound, even if there is only one break, because the exposed blood vessels, nerves and muscle are in great danger of infection. There is often a lot of bleeding.

HOW TO TELL IF BONES ARE BROKEN

The arm or leg is swollen in the area of the fracture.

The area is black and blue. (may not show at first).

Finger pressure over the fracture causes severe pain.

You can't move the hurt part without pain.

It may look deformed. (If the bones are not displaced, it will *not* look deformed, but may still be fractured).

WHAT NOT TO DO WHEN BONES ARE BROKEN

A fracture is one emergency that almost never needs to be cared for quickly. So unless it's absolutely necessary for safety, don't move victim until ambulance comes. If you *must* move him, see directions (page 55).

- Don't pull victim into the back seat of a car. If there is a back injury this can be especially harmful.

- Don't let him stand or sit up or move the injured part.

- If neck is injured, *don't* put pillow under head. Block head on both sides so it doesn't move.

- Don't try to set bones if medical help is delayed. Just apply splints before moving victim (see page 70).

BROKEN BONES

WHAT TO DO ABOUT BROKEN BONES

- Stop serious bleeding by hand pressure directly over wound. If no gauze or clean cloth is handy, use the heel of your bare hand.

- Check mouth and throat to see that airway is open. Give artificial respiration if needed.

- Cut clothing away *gently* so injured part is not moved. Do *not* pull if clothes stick.

- Leave patient lying down. Just cover him to keep him warm.

- If skin is broken or bone sticks out, apply clean dressing but no antiseptic.

- If skin is not broken, cover with cool compresses (cool, damp cloths). If possible, make a splint.

MAKING A SPLINT

MATERIALS:

Use anything rigid enough to give broken part constant support and stop broken ends from grinding together. Boards, sticks, rifle barrels, umbrellas, broomstick, baseball bat, tightly rolled magazines or newspapers are all good do-it-yourself splints. Pad with something soft to shield injured part. Splint should be long enough to go beyond the nearest joint in both directions and to prevent motion. For example: For leg, the splints should include knee and ankle joints. (See Bandaging, page 103).

BROKEN BONES

TREATING BROKEN BONES

HEAD AND FACE

Raise lower jaw gently to normal position and support with broad bandage under chin tied as shown. If patient vomits or bleeds from mouth, remove bandage at once. Turn head to side, support jaw gently with hand and replace bandage when bleeding or vomiting stops.

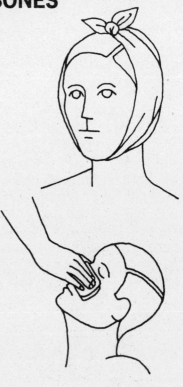

NOSE

Don't splint broken nose. Press sides of nose together between thumb and index finger for a few minutes if there is bleeding. Press cold cloth over nose as patient holds head back slightly. See doctor promptly to avoid deformity.

SKULL (Head Injury)

No head injury is unimportant. See a doctor for *any* head injury right away. You can walk around with a concussion without knowing it.

- Keep injured person warm and lying down. Keeping quiet is only way to reduce internal bleeding.

- *Give no food or liquid.*

- Turn head to side to let secretions escape from mouth.

BROKEN BONES

- If scalp is bleeding, press gauze *lightly* in place without pressure to avoid driving bone fragments into brain.
- *Do not move* person unless absolutely necessary for safety. If you must move the person, support head with pads at sides to prevent motion.

Watch for these danger signs:

- Bleeding from nose and ears.
- State of confusion or amnesia.
- May collapse from later internal bleeding.
- Blurring vision or dizziness.
- Headaches.
- Mental disturbances such as changes of personality or permanent coma.

NECK OR BACK

Any movement of head or back can be fatal or cause lasting paralysis.

- Don't move or lift patient.
- Don't bend or twist head or body in any direction.
- Don't put a pillow under head.
- Don't give water or cigarettes.
- Don't pull him out of wrecked car unless there is danger of fire or explosion.
- Don't rush him to hospital. Leave him where he is until the doctor comes.

If the victim cannot move his fingers readily, or if there is tingling or numbness around his shoulder, *his neck may be broken.*

If he can move his fingers but not his feet or toes, or if he has tingling or numbness in his legs, or pain when he tries to move, *his back or neck may be broken.*

72

BROKEN BONES

FOREARM OR WRIST

Put patient on his back.
Place forearm at right angle across chest.
Put padded splints from elbow to back of fingers.
Tie splint in place with bandages above and below break.
Adjust necktie sling so that fingertips are 3 or 4 inches above elbow. (See pages 107, 112.)

UPPER ARM

Put forearm across chest, palm side in.
Put splint outside arm from below elbow to above shoulder.
Tie with two cloth strips above and below fracture.
Support forearm with necktie sling.
Bind upper arm to body with towel or cloth around splint and chest.
Tie under other arm. (See page 112.)

ELBOW

If elbow is bent, don't straighten it out.
Put arm in sling and bind it firmly to body.
If arm and elbow are straight, leave them that way.
Just put a splint on inside of arm from fingertips to armpit.
Tie above and below *without* touching elbow.
For comfort don't push splint too close to armpit. (See page 114.)

LOWER LEG: KNEE TO ANKLE

Leave victim's shoes on. This makes traction easier and decreases the chance of displacing the bones even more.
Hold foot firmly and pull slowly to put in normal position.
If alone, tie feet together after leg is in position.
(Otherwise hold leg in position while helper fixes splint.)
Be careful, as jagged bones may break through skin or cut blood vessels.

BROKEN BONES

THIGH

Treat for shock (see page 36) and get doctor quickly.
Injured leg may be shortened so put one hand *under* heel, the other over instep.
Steady leg and pull gently into normal position.
Fix 7 broad, long bandages and use small stick to push them under hollows of knees and back.
Put 4" to 6" wide splint on the outer part of the leg from arm-pit to heel.
Put splint on inner part of leg from crotch to heel.
Tie together.
(If no splints are available, pad well and use uninjured leg as splint.)

KNEECAP

Straighten leg gently and rest it on board under leg.
Put extra padding under knee and ankle.
Tie above and below kneecap.

ANKLE

Extend pillow or blanket splint
well beyond heel as shown.

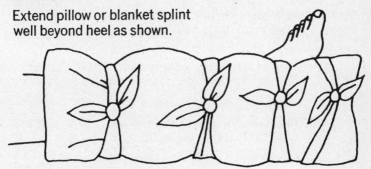

FOOT OR TOES

Put splint under sole of foot and tie snugly but not tightly. (See page 106.)

BROKEN BONES

COLLAR BONE

Patient usually cannot raise arm above shoulder. Injured shoulder is lower when arms hang down. Put arm in sling, leaving fingertips exposed. Adjust to comfortable height (See page 112). Tie arm to body with towel or cloth over sling.

RIBS

Pain with movement, breathing or coughing usually means a fracture. *Don't bind too tightly* because broken rib-ends can puncture lung.

- Put broad pad over break. Then tie broad cloth strip around chest, making knot over pad.

- Tie second knot for firm support.

- *If patient coughs up blood, froth or bright red blood, do not apply tighter bandages. Give first aid for shock until doctor arrives.*

PELVIS

This is serious. Broken bones in this area may damage important organs. Don't move patient if help is on the way.

- Bandage ankles and knees together keeping legs straight or bent.
- If patient *must* be moved, slide broad bandage under hollow of back and work under hips. Tie or pin snugly, not tightly.
- Put patient on his back on a board (a flat door will do).
- If you do not have a board or door, a sheet or blanket can be used as a sling for carrying the patient.

See Moving an Injured Person, page 55.

REMEMBER
THE EIGHT BASIC LIFE SAVING
STEPS IN FIRST AID
SEE INSIDE FRONT COVER FOR DETAILS

1. Verify breathing. If stopped or very weak, give mouth-to-mouth rescue breathing *at once*.

2. Do not move victim unless absolutely necessary for safety (fire or other danger to life).
   Keep him lying flat on level surface.

3. Stop bleeding. Apply pressure *directly* over wound with a compress or the heel of your hand if that is all you have.

4. Keep injured person warm (but not hot) to prevent shock.

5. Give nothing by mouth if injured person is unconscious or semi-conscious.

6. Calm victim by staying calm yourself.

7. Obtain information for doctor: victim's name, address, nature of injuries.

8. Get medical help fast. Stay with victim. If you can, have someone else telephone for help.

REMEMBER
EMERGENCY NUMBERS ON INSIDE BACK COVER

WOUNDS/CUTS/BRUISES

MAJOR WOUNDS AND CUTS

Call doctor AT ONCE for all accidents listed.

- Don't move patient unless absolutely necessary.
- Stop bleeding by applying pressure directly over wound (see page 25).
- Keep patient covered, warm, to treat shock.
- Keep breathing passage clear.
- Don't give stimulants.
- Cover wound with sterile dressing.
- Unless told to, *don't* use antiseptics.

DEEP CUTS

Do not try to clean wound. Chances of infection are small.

The edges of cuts from sharp objects like knives, razors or broken glass are usually smooth, not jagged. Bleeding may be heavy, and arteries, nerves or tendons may be damaged.

Control bleeding by pressing hand over clean cloth until doctor arrives. Cover with sterile gauze or adhesive bandage. Do not remove anything from the wound (for example, a knife or glass.)

EXCEPTION: If the wound is to the chest or stomach, the object should be removed as soon as possible. This is because the patient could suffer injuries to lungs or intestines from his own breathing movements.

JAGGED CUTS

Jagged cuts are caused by blunt instruments or falls against sharp objects. The danger of infection is greater than in a clean, deep cut, and healing is usually slower. Bleeding is seldom heavy, however nerves or tendons may be damaged. Cover with sterile gauze or adhesive bandage.

WOUNDS/CUTS/BRUISES

PUNCTURE WOUNDS

May be caused by gunshot, nails, fishhooks, ice picks, knives. Never remove a wood splinter that is deeply buried. It may be plugging injured vessels, and removal may cause fatal bleeding. *Puncture wounds may look harmless on the surface and cause little bleeding on the outside. However, serious injury and infection may result.*

GUNSHOT WOUNDS

Treat like any puncture wound. Always suspect broken bones and internal hemorrhage or injury to vital organs because no one knows where the bullet has gone inside the body. If an extremity has been shot, splint it before the patient has to be moved. Report any gunshot injuries to the police.

DEEP CHEST WOUNDS

When an object such as a knife, ice pick or bullet goes through the chest wall, you hear a hissing "sucking" sound of air going in and out of the wound. The lung will totally collapse and death may result unless the victim gets first aid at once.

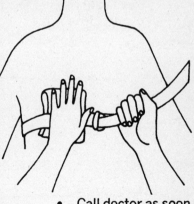

- Put thick pad or sterile gauze over wound only when the victim breathes OUT (not in). By doing this, the victim *himself* will refill his collapsed lung the next time he breathes in.

- Hold pad firmly in place with adhesive tape or tightly drawn belt. *Important:* make sure no air leaks in. Bandage *must* be airtight.

- Call doctor as soon as possible.

WOUNDS/CUTS/BRUISES

ABDOMINAL INJURIES

Little can be done about internal injuries until a doctor examines them.

- *Give patient nothing by mouth, not even water.*
- Put sterile dressing over wound to bring edges together and stop bleeding.

EXPOSED INTESTINES

- *Do not attempt to push organs back into place.*
- Cover exposed intestines with sterile dressing or clean cloth which must be kept moist.
- Get to a hospital as soon as possible, where victim has only chance to recover.

In the meantime:

- *Give patient nothing by mouth.*
- Keep patient flat on back with knees bent. Support knees by putting coat or blanket under them.
- Keep patient quiet and resting.

REMEMBER
EMERGENCY NUMBERS ON INSIDE BACK COVER

WOUNDS/CUTS/BRUISES

MINOR WOUNDS, CUTS AND BRUISES

- Wash gently with soap and water, using sterile or clean gauze or cotton.

- Pick out small bits of coarse dirt with tweezers. (Before using tweezers: pass them through a match or gas flame, but don't burn the person).

- Black and blue marks may mean further injury such as broken bones or bleeding. Cover with cool compresses (cool, damp cloths). Do not try to move the part.

- If redness, pain, or swelling gets worse, or cut has been touched by manure or excrement, *call doctor.*

- A minor cut can lead to lockjaw if the tetanus germ gets into the wound. If person has not been recently immunized, he should see a doctor and get a tetanus shot. This also holds true for puncture wounds and animal bites.

BRUISES (Black Eye)

Apply ice bag or cold compresses immediately to reduce tissue bleeding. After a day or so, apply hot moist towels wrung out.

SPLINTERS

Clean skin with soap and water or alcohol.

Sterilize a needle and tweezers by holding tips of both in flame a few seconds. After cooling, press firmly against the skin with the needle, stroking it toward place splinter entered. Grasp loosened end of splinter with tweezers and pull it out at same angle it entered skin.

80

WOUNDS/CUTS/BRUISES

BOILS

Boils in the diabetic person can be serious. Do not squeeze boils or pimples as this may spread infection or lead to blood poisoning and abscess. Keep affected area free from pressure or friction. Help boils heal faster by applying hot, moist wash-cloths as frequently as possible.

BLISTERS

Leave blisters alone. Opening them invites infection. Keep blisters clean and they will heal by themselves in most cases.

FISHHOOKS IN FLESH

Do nothing if fishhook went into face or skin around the eyes.

If medical help is not nearby, press down on shank of hook until bared and push through skin. Cut off barbed end with pliers or clippers. Remove shaft of hook. Wash wound with soap and water, encouraging bleeding. Cover wound.

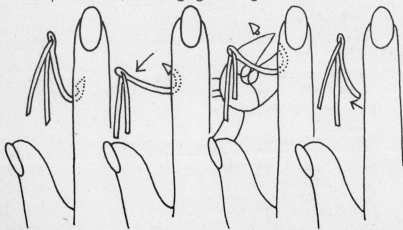

WOUNDS/CUTS/BRUISES

ALTERNATE METHOD OF HOOK REMOVAL

Make a loop of ordinary string about 18 inches long. Slip the loop over the shank of the hook, wind the ends around your own right index finger. Place the patient's finger on a firm surface, push down on the shank to disengage the barb. Jerk the string quickly to pull the hook out.

If you can get to a doctor within a few hours, leave hook in place. The doctor can remove it painlessly.

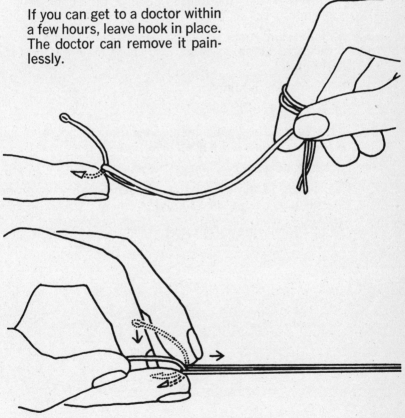

See doctor as soon as possible as victim may need tetanus shot.

SPRAINS/STRAINS/ DISLOCATIONS

SPRAINS, STRAINS AND DISLOCATIONS

SPRAINS

Sprains happen when the joint is pushed into action beyond its usual limits.

Signs of a sprain: rapid swelling; pain in joint; tenderness to touch; black and blue discoloration. These may not show for several hours.

- Relieve pain by resting joint.
- Raise it so it gets less blood.
- Bandage it to prevent unnecessary motion for 24 hours. (An elastic bandage is a good idea.)
- Loosen bandage if swelling gets worse.
- Use ice bag for first few hours to keep swelling down and ease pain. Severe sprains should be splinted.
- After a day or so, use hot compresses.

SPRAINS/STRAINS/ DISLOCATIONS

ANKLE SPRAIN

- *Never walk with a sprained ankle. It may be broken.*

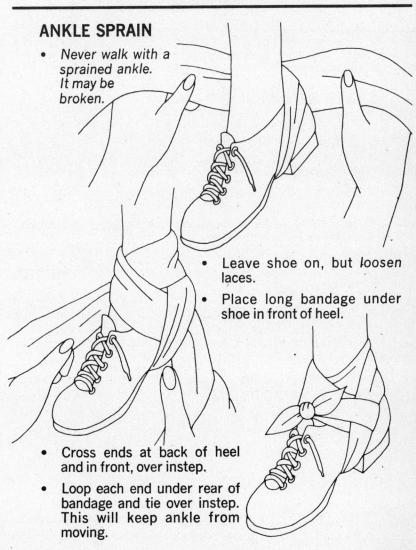

- Leave shoe on, but *loosen* laces.
- Place long bandage under shoe in front of heel.

- Cross ends at back of heel and in front, over instep.
- Loop each end under rear of bandage and tie over instep. This will keep ankle from moving.

SPRAINS/STRAINS/ DISLOCATIONS

STRAINS

Strains happen when muscles are "overworked." A "charley horse" is a strain.

HOW TO HANDLE A STRAIN

- Rest the strained muscle by not moving the part that hurts.

- At first use cold ice packs on the strain. After a couple of hours applying heat is best.

- After a few hours put an electric heating pad or hot water bottle on the hurting spot *unless* the pain is in the calf. If there is *calf pain*, put *ice pack* on sore spot to lessen hemorrhage and swelling in leg.

- Call your doctor.

BACK STRAINS

Low back strain is caused mainly by lifting things the wrong way or carrying things the wrong way. Avoid a sway back position. Keep back straight, feet flat on floor close to whatever you're lifting.

Always *bend* down with your knees and ankles to lift something (keeping back straight).

SPRAINS/STRAINS/ DISLOCATIONS

DISLOCATIONS

A dislocation happens when a bone slips out of its normal position in the joint. Ligaments around the joint may be torn or loosened. Symptoms are like those of fracture: pain; swelling; tenderness; an abnormal look; limited ability to move, or complete inability to move.

- Don't try to straighten out joint or force bone back in place except for jaw, finger or toes.
- Suspect possible fractures.
- Keep weight off injured part and support it.
- Apply ice bag or cloths wrung out in cold water.
- Call a doctor.
- Apply a splint.

JAW DISLOCATION

Symptoms: Lower jaw sags down and person can't close mouth.

- Get a metal rod, spoon handle or similar object to use as a bit.
- Wrap object with cloth to make it soft.
- Sit patient in chair and face him.
- Close jaw around the cloth-covered bit.
- Get to a doctor as soon as possible.

SPRAINS/STRAINS/ DISLOCATIONS

FINGER OR TOE DISLOCATION

- Grasp with one hand on *each* side of dislocated joint.

- Slowly pull free end of toe or finger straight until it snaps back into place. *Do not use a lot of force. Never* pull dislocated joint if open wound is near it.

- *Splint by taping injured part to next finger or toe—* See page 106.

- Small fractures are often associated with dislocations so fingers and toes should be seen by a doctor and x-rayed.

- Call a doctor.

FIRST AID IS NOT A SUBSTITUTE FOR MEDICAL HELP. ALWAYS SEND FOR THE DOCTOR AS QUICKLY AS POSSIBLE.

REMEMBER
THE EIGHT BASIC LIFE SAVING
STEPS IN FIRST AID
SEE INSIDE FRONT COVER FOR DETAILS

1. Verify breathing. If stopped or very weak, give mouth-to-mouth rescue breathing *at once.*

2. Do not move victim unless absolutely necessary for safety (fire or other danger to life).
   Keep him lying flat on level surface.

3. Stop bleeding. Apply pressure *directly* over wound with a compress or the heel of your hand if that is all you have.

4. Keep injured person warm (but not hot) to prevent shock.

5. Give nothing by mouth if injured person is unconscious or semi-conscious.

6. Calm victim by staying calm yourself.

7. Obtain information for doctor: victim's name, address, nature of injuries.

8. Get medical help fast. Stay with victim. If you can, have someone else telephone for help.

REMEMBER
EMERGENCY NUMBERS ON INSIDE BACK COVER

BITES/STINGS

ANIMAL BITES

RABIES CAN KILL.

Most bites are from healthy animals. But *bites from dogs, cats, skunks, foxes, bats and other animals can cause rabies.* Rabies is a disease that kills UNLESS it is treated.

FIRST AID FOR ALL ANIMAL BITES

Even bites from healthy animals can cause serious infections. Treat animal bites quickly. If skin is broken, see doctor at once.

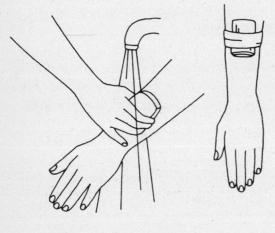

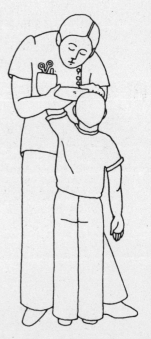

Wash *thoroughly* with soap and water. Use *running water* if you can.

Cover with a sterile dressing, such as a gauze pad.

Always see a doctor if bite goes through the skin as you may need a tetanus shot.

89

BITES/STINGS

- *If the animal acts strangely or attacks for no reason,* it may have rabies. Be suspicious of *any* bat bite.

- Do not shoot animal in the head or crush its head as examination of the animals head is necessary to determine if it had rabies.

- Try to catch the animal so a doctor can examine it. If it acts dangerously, *take care not to get bitten yourself. Get help if necessary.* Do not kill the animal. It should be captured and kept in captivity for 2 weeks.

- *If it is a pet, find out who owns it.* The owner will know if his pet has had shots to prevent rabies.

TREATMENT FOR RABIES

- If the animal has rabies, *the victim can be protected from the disease by a series of injections.*

- Report the bite immediately. *Give all the information you can to doctor. He can decide if the treatments are needed.*

HUMAN BITES

People carry germs in their mouths.
A human bite may cause as severe a local infection as an animal bite. *Treat a human bite with the same first aid as an animal bite.*

BITES/STINGS

INSECT BITES AND STINGS

Most bites and stings are harmless, although they may hurt or itch. Do NOT scratch because scratching can cause infection.

Stings from bees, wasps, hornets and yellow jackets.

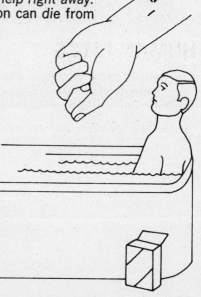

- Some people get *very* sick from just one sting if they are allergic to it. *If you know the victim has this allergy, get medical help right away.* Such a person can *die* from stings.

- Get *the stinger out* if it is left in the skin. Scrape it out with a clean tweezers. (Boil tweezers or clean with alcohol). *Do NOT squeeze it* or you will squeeze more painful venom into the sting.

- Treat the sting to relieve pain. (See page 93.)

  If you are stung many times, take a "soda bath": Pour a small box of *baking soda (bicarbonate of soda)* into a tub of warm *(not hot)* water. Get into the tub and soak.

91

BITES/STINGS

SPIDER BITES

WATCH OUT FOR THE BLACK WIDOW SPIDER.

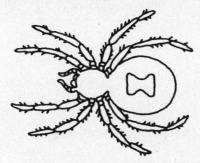

Shiny black, ½ inch long. Red or orange spot, shaped like hourglass, on underside.

- Spider bites are rare. *Most spiders are harmless.*

- *The bite of the black widow spider causes severe pain. It feels like a needle prick and leaves two tiny red marks.*

- The pain may spread. Later, there are severe muscle cramps and pain in the abdomen. *If these signs show up, call a doctor.* Save the spider to show him if you can. *Don't wait for the pain,* see a doctor as soon as possible.

- While you wait for the doctor, do this:

Wash bite with soap and water. Put on a paste made of baking soda and water. Watch for signs of shock.

BROWN RECLUSE SPIDER

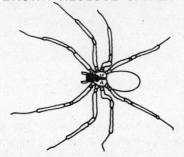

The brown recluse spider is also very poisonous. It is common, lives in dark corners indoors and out, has a dark violin-shaped mark extending back from its eyes.

92

BITES/STINGS

HOW TO HELP STOP PAIN AND ITCH FROM INSECT BITES

- *Cold helps.* Put ice or a cool wet cloth on the bite, or hold it under cold water.

- *Baking soda helps.* Mix some with a little water, then spread it on the bite. *Or mix household ammonia with water,* then wipe it on the bite.

- *Calamine lotion or rubbing alcohol* on the bite help stop itching.

- Avoid infection. *Do not scratch* bites and stings.

FIRST AID IS NOT A SUBSTITUTE FOR MEDICAL HELP. ALWAYS SEND FOR THE DOCTOR AS QUICKLY AS POSSIBLE.

REMEMBER
THE EIGHT BASIC LIFE SAVING
STEPS IN FIRST AID
SEE INSIDE FRONT COVER FOR DETAILS

1. Verify breathing. If stopped or very weak, give mouth-to-mouth rescue breathing *at once.*

2. Do not move victim unless absolutely necessary for safety (fire or other danger to life).
   Keep him lying flat on level surface.

3. Stop bleeding. Apply pressure *directly* over wound with a compress or the heel of your hand if that is all you have.

4. Keep injured person warm (but not hot) to prevent shock.

5. Give nothing by mouth if injured person is unconscious or semi-conscious.

6. Calm victim by staying calm yourself.

7. Obtain information for doctor: victim's name, address, nature of injuries.

8. Get medical help fast. Stay with victim. If you can, have someone else telephone for help.

REMEMBER
EMERGENCY NUMBERS ON INSIDE BACK COVER

BITES/STINGS

TICK BITES

Some ticks can cause serious illness. Treat at once. Under a magnifying glass, ticks look like this:

Ticks dig into the skin and are hard to get loose.

If you camp or hike where there are ticks, look for them on clothes and body every day. *Get rid of them right away.* Wear clothes that protect your entire body, *especially* the arms and legs.

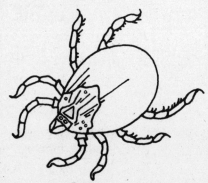

TO GET RID OF TICKS:

- *Brush oil* (cooking oil; mineral oil or machine oil) *or nail polish over the tick* on the skin. The tick may let loose right away. If not, *brush* again and wait half an hour. Then use tweezers to get its head out.

- *Wash the spot well with soap and water after* the tick is out.

- *Save the tick to show a doctor.* He can decide if you need treatment to prevent disease carried by ticks.

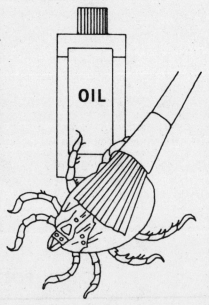

BITES/STINGS

SNAKE BITE

If there is much swelling, the bite marks may be hidden.

Severe swelling or instant sharp pain usually means the snake is poisonous.

Most snakes in the United States are not poisonous. The poisonous snakes are rattlers, copperheads, moccasins and the rare coral snake in the South.

Most poisonous snakes leave two *puncture marks (holes)* in the skin when they bite.

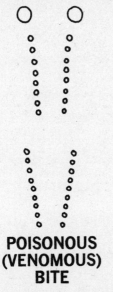

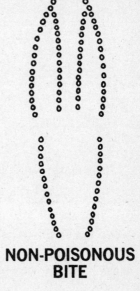

POISONOUS (VENOMOUS) BITE

NON-POISONOUS BITE

The puncture marks are caused by the fangs. Poison enters the holes from the fangs. You may also see rows of tiny scratches that are tooth marks.

Bite marks like this are usually *not* poisonous. NOTICE that there are no puncture marks here.

BITES/STINGS

WHAT TO DO FOR POISONOUS BITES
(and bites you are not sure of)

Place a tourniquet between the bite and the heart. Loosen it every 15 minutes.

Get victim to doctor immediately for an antivenin shot.

If you are in an isolated area where no doctor is available, give the shot yourself.

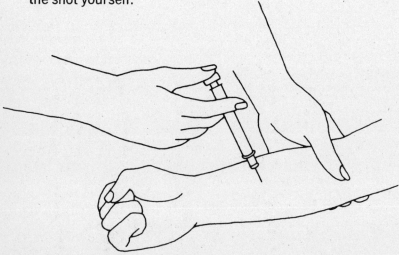

Keep the victim as still as possible.

Moving around spreads the poison through the body faster. Have him lie down quietly.

Do NOT give stimulants (coffee, whiskey, any alcoholic drink). They also spread the poison faster.

Get medical help as quickly as you can.

If there is no phone to call for help, *carry the victim* to the nearest phone or doctor.

97

BITES/STINGS

Get the victim to a doctor

Use a stretcher if you have someone to help.

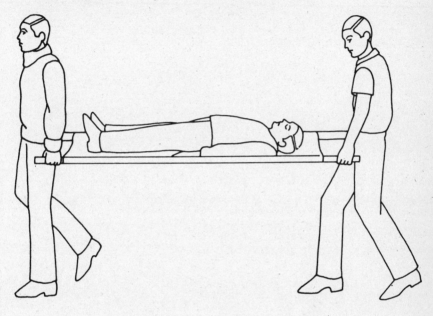

You can make a stretcher from two shirts and two poles.

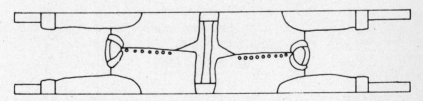

A sheet or blanket can also be used as a sling for carrying the patient.

BITES/STINGS

Carry the victim if you are alone. Let the bitten part hang lower than the rest of the body to slow down the spread of poison.

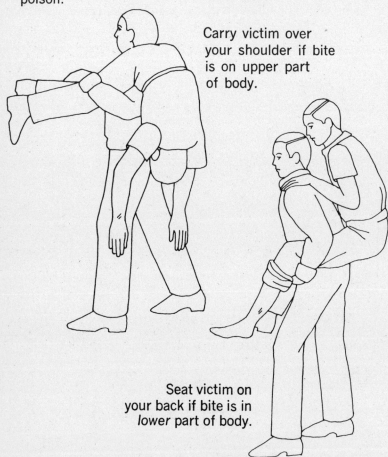

Carry victim over your shoulder if bite is on upper part of body.

Seat victim on your back if bite is in *lower* part of body.

See *Moving an Injured Person,* page 55.

Poisonous snake bites must be treated at once. If medical help is hours away, use the INCISION-SUCTION METHOD.

BITES/STINGS

INCISION-SUCTION METHOD
FOR POISONOUS SNAKE BITES

Use this method only if NO medical help is available quickly.

Use for bites on foot, leg, arm or hand. It cannot harm you and it may save the victim's life.

1. *Apply a tourniquet* (see page 29). Place tourniquet *between* the wound and the heart, a few inches above the bite.

2. *Make small cuts over puncture holes to cause bleeding.*

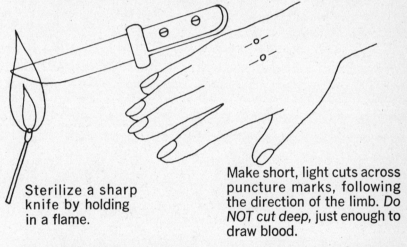

Sterilize a sharp knife by holding in a flame.

Make short, light cuts across puncture marks, following the direction of the limb. *Do NOT cut deep,* just enough to draw blood.

3. *Suck out blood coming from cuts.* Continue for at least one hour, resting as needed.

Use a suction cup if you have one, otherwise suck the blood by mouth. The poison only acts through the bloodstream, so *sucking it out will not harm you.*

4. *Have bite treated by a doctor as soon as possible.*

100

BITES/STINGS

MORE ON SNAKE BITES

How to treat non-poisonous snake bites:

Treat like any other skin wound to stop infection:

- *Clean* well with soap and warm water.
- *Cover* with a sterile dressing, such as a gauze pad.
- *See your doctor* and get a tetanus shot.

Play it safe and avoid snake bites:

- *Wear high leather boots* to protect your ankles when you are in snake country.
- Walk carefully through places where snakes may be hiding.

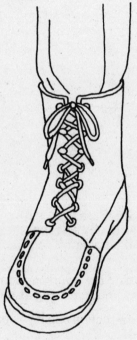

Be prepared for snake bites.

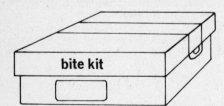

bite kit

Take along a snake-bite kit if you camp or hike where poisonous snakes are common. You can buy such kits in drugstores. They contain basic equipment such as tourniquet, antiseptic, suction bulb and sometimes antivenom.

REMEMBER
THE EIGHT BASIC LIFE SAVING
STEPS IN FIRST AID
SEE INSIDE FRONT COVER FOR DETAILS

1. Verify breathing. If stopped or very weak, give mouth-to-mouth rescue breathing *at once.*

2. Do not move victim unless absolutely necessary for safety (fire or other danger to life).
   Keep him lying flat on level surface.

3. Stop bleeding. Apply pressure *directly* over wound with a compress or the heel of your hand if that is all you have.

4. Keep injured person warm (but not hot) to prevent shock.

5. Give nothing by mouth if injured person is unconscious or semi-conscious.

6. Calm victim by staying calm yourself.

7. Obtain information for doctor: victim's name, address, nature of injuries.

8. Get medical help fast. Stay with victim. If you can, have someone else telephone for help.

REMEMBER
EMERGENCY NUMBERS ON INSIDE BACK COVER

BANDAGING

BANDAGING AND BANDAGES

Don't try to make a professional bandage in an emergency unless you have done it before. Remember, the doctor will make a new one when he gets there. Your job as a first-aider is to stop any bleeding, keep dirt from the wound, and protect the injury.

1. Begin by applying sterile gauze compresses big enough to cover the wound. Place bandage (pictures show how on pages 105 to 114) over the compress.

2. Fit the bandage firmly but *not* tightly.

3. If you see any swelling, blueness, or edge of bandage cutting into skin, loosen bandage. Wound can swell and make bandage so tight it cuts off circulation.

BANDAGING

**TYPES OF BANDAGES TO KEEP
IN YOUR FIRST AID KIT:**

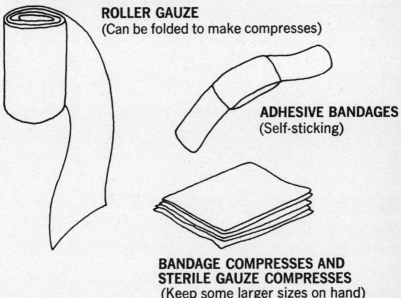

ROLLER GAUZE
(Can be folded to make compresses)

ADHESIVE BANDAGES
(Self-sticking)

**BANDAGE COMPRESSES AND
STERILE GAUZE COMPRESSES**
(Keep some larger sizes on hand)

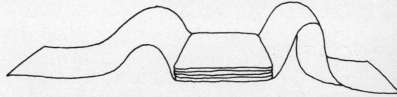

**Elastic type bandages and self-sticking (adhesive) compresses
are the easiest to use.**

In emergency, use the cleanest cloth available (sheets, pillow
cases, napkins, towels) if there are no sterile bandages.

**NEVER USE FLUFFY ABSORBENT COTTON DIRECTLY ON A
BLEEDING WOUND.**

104

BANDAGING

TRIANGULAR BANDAGE (CRAVAT)

How to make one:

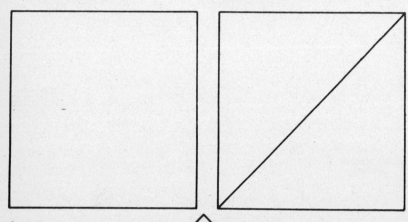

1. Cut a 40-inch square out of a sheet of cloth.

2. Then cut into 2 triangle bandages.

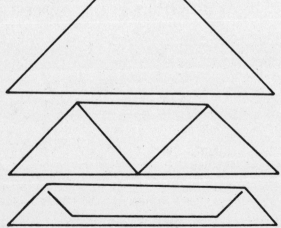

3. To make a "cravat" roll triangle as shown.

BANDAGING

HOW TO BANDAGE

Finger bandage:

Wrap and tie one end of gauze at wrist.

Wind bandage in spirals down finger, then back to wrist; tie at wrist.

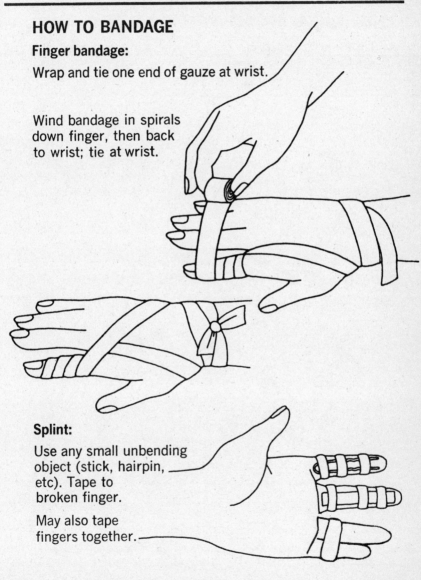

Splint:

Use any small unbending object (stick, hairpin, etc). Tape to broken finger.

May also tape fingers together.

BANDAGING

Hand or Wrist:

Tie at wrist, wrap criss-cross over hand and tape at wrist again.

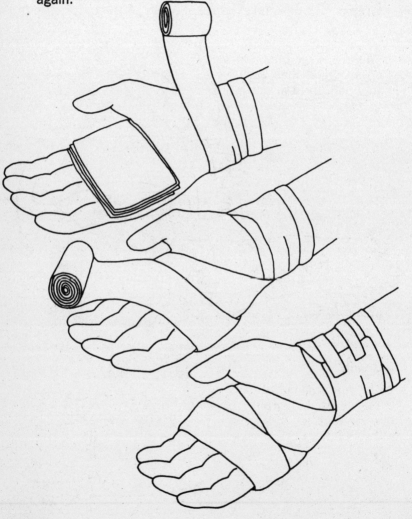

BANDAGING

Arm or Leg:

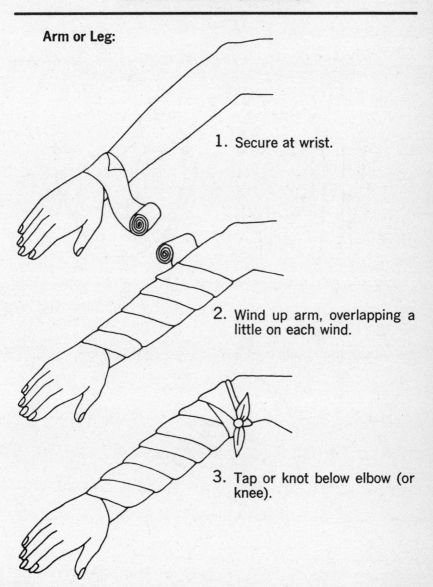

1. Secure at wrist.

2. Wind up arm, overlapping a little on each wind.

3. Tap or knot below elbow (or knee).

BANDAGING

Eye:

Cravat should be comfortable, not tight.

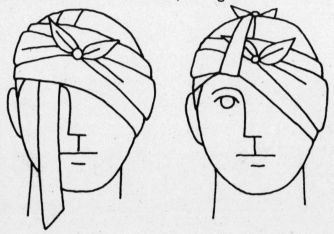

Ear or Head:

Cover wound with compress. Tie cravat over it.

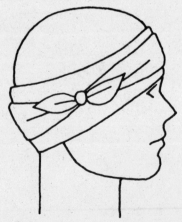

BANDAGING

Scalp or Forehead:

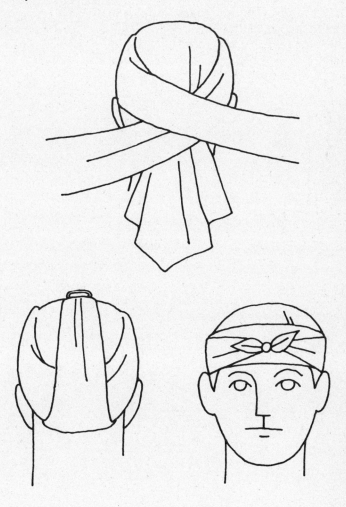

BANDAGING

Palm of Hand:

Put compress directly over wound, then wrap cravat around hand. Leave thumb out.

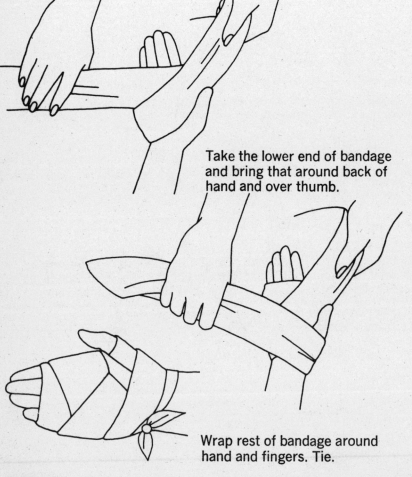

Take the lower end of bandage and bring that around back of hand and over thumb.

Wrap rest of bandage around hand and fingers. Tie.

BANDAGING

Arm Sling:

Use triangle bandage. Tie behind neck. Check that knot isn't pressing on spine. Pin at elbow. If forearm is injured, raise hand a little above elbow.

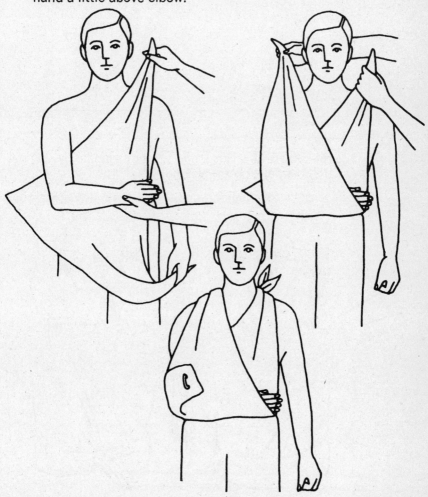

BANDAGING

Body Bandage:

Roll longest side of triangle bandage up part way.

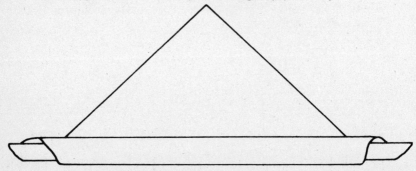

Tie the rolled part at waist. Place point of triangle over shoulder, so that bandage covers wound.

Tie extra cloth to shoulder point, and tie that part around body.

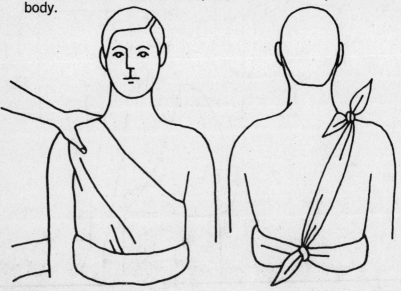

BANDAGING

Elbow (or Knee) Compress:

(Use elastic bandage if you have one, or a cravat at least 8 inches wide.)

Put compress over wound. Bend elbow. Place middle of bandage over the elbow (or knee). Wrap and tie.

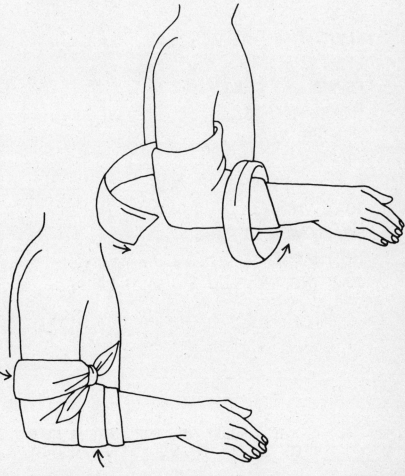

GENERAL EMERGENCY

GENERAL PROBLEMS

    APPENDICITIS

    DIARRHEA

    DRUG EMERGENCY

    EARACHE

    EMOTIONAL EMERGENCIES

    EYE PROBLEMS

    FEVER AND CHILLS

    HEART ATTACK

    HEMORRHOIDS

    HICCOUGHS

    PREGNANCY EMERGENCIES

    SORE THROAT

    SWALLOWED OBJECTS

    TOOTHACHE

    VOMITING, NAUSEA, STOMACH PAINS

FIRST AID IS NOT A SUBSTITUTE FOR MEDICAL HELP.
ALWAYS SEND FOR THE DOCTOR AS QUICKLY AS POSSIBLE.

GENERAL EMERGENCY

APPENDICITIS

The appendix is usually on the right side of the abdomen below the level of your waist, but the pain may start elsewhere. If the appendix is inflamed, it must be removed because it may rupture and cause peritonitis. Appendicitis occurs more often in younger people.

Never put a hot water bottle on victim if you think the problem may be appendicitis.

Never give a suspected appendicitis victim any food or drink.

Call the doctor.

GENERAL EMERGENCY

DIARRHEA

Frequent soft or liquid bowel movements can mean a great many things. If it continues or recurs, or if there's blood in the movement, call your doctor right away. The main causes of prolonged diarrhea are spoiled food, virus infections, and laxative foods like bran, figs, and prunes.

If diarrhea occurs **without** pain, vomiting, fever or blood in the movement, here's what to do:

- Eat nothing for up to 24 hours.

- If thirsty, chew on ice cubes or crushed ice, take frequent sips of water, weak tea, ginger ale or clear broth. You may need to stay on clear liquids for 24 or 48 hours.

- Once you bring diarrhea under control, gradually start on foods like salted crackers, dry or melba toast, gelatin desserts, mashed or baked potato, white rice, cooked or dry rice cereals, jellied consomme. Later you can add a soft-boiled or poached egg, cooked carrots or peas, a thin slice of white meat chicken or turkey. *If diarrhea recurs with loss of appetite or nausea* after any of these foods, stop taking food or liquids for four to six hours and gradually go back to clear liquids and foods listed above.

- Don't take any raw fruits or vegtables, coffee, spices (other than salt) or rich, fatty or fried foods.

- While you can get many remedies without a prescription, it is generally a good idea to talk to your doctor first.

DRUG EMERGENCIES

If you think a person may be under the influence of drugs:

- Be calm and reassuring.

- Do not argue or try to reason with person.

- Call doctor or hospital as soon as possible.

- See pages 120 and 121.

117

GENERAL EMERGENCY

EARACHE

Call your doctor whenever an earache continues for an hour or two without stopping or becoming less painful. *Don't* put anything in your ear such as cotton swab, hairpin, paper clip, fingernail or any ointment or drops. This may do harm or interfere with doctor's examination.

THINGS IN THE EAR

If insect, pebble, stone, seed, or any object gets caught in the ear, *don't* try to wash it out with oil or water. Don't try to remove it with any object *including* your fingernail. Call your doctor and let him do it.

WHAT TO DO FOR EARACHE

1. Apply a hot water bottle or heating pad to ear.

2. Chew gum or yawn a lot. (Especially when short earache is caused by a change of altitude, as in an airplane.)

3. Use nose drops in the *nose.* This sometimes helps open a clogged ear. Be sure the nose drops were prescribed for you by your doctor when you had a cold, and have not changed color.

4. Take aspirin or any pain reliever prescribed in the past.

5. If an insect gets in the ear, you can often get it to crawl out by holding a bright light close to the ear.

GENERAL EMERGENCY

WHEN TO CALL THE DOCTOR

- If you can't hear normally.
- If you have pain in the ear.
- If you have a feeling of fullness in the ear.
- If you're dizzy.
- If you have ringing in the ears or strange sounds like buzzing, thumping, roaring or whistling.
- If you have a discharge coming from the ear.

EMOTIONAL EMERGENCIES

THREATENED SUICIDE

Take suicide threats seriously except from people who use such threats daily as "slang." Every year 25,000 people succeed in committing suicide. Five million Americans now alive have at one time or another tried to do this. Suicide is the ninth leading cause of death in the United States. It is not true that most people who threaten suicide aren't serious.

PEOPLE MOST LIKELY TO COMMIT SUICIDE

Anyone who is depressed or hopeless, feels worthless, or loses in interest in things which previously interested him.

Anyone who is impulsive and doesn't give much thought to consequences of his acts. (Such people are often alcoholic).

Anyone who wants to kill himself for drama or to serve some purpose. (Such people are most often young and immature).

Adolescents are particularly capable of suicide for these reasons.

Anyone in constant pain or who believes he has an incurable illness.

119

GENERAL EMERGENCY

DANGEROUS OR VIOLENT BEHAVIOR

Violent behavior is most likely to follow a period of strange, threatening, angry behavior. It can, however, come without warning. The people involved are often mentally or physically ill.

Common causes are: confused states resulting from high fever, other illness or medications, certain rare types of epilepsy, panic states, paranoid schizophrenic reactions, the manic phase of a manic-depressive illness, hallucinogenic drugs, LSD, alcoholism or recent or repeated head injuries.

WHAT TO DO

1. Keep calm.

2. Don't argue, reason, restrain or fight back.

3. Get away as quickly as possible, taking any children with you and warning any endangered adults.

4. Call doctor as soon as you're safely away and possibly the police.

DISORIENTATION OR MENTAL CONFUSION

Mental or physical illness or intoxication causes loss of contact with reality. A person may be dazed or confused as to who he is, who you are, where he is, what time, day or year it is. He may be unaware of his confusion or subject to hallucinations, illusions or delusions. Delirium is a state of total confusion, no contact with reality at all.

Some common causes are: fever, alcoholic or other forms of intoxication, many kinds of medication in normal or excessive dosage, head injury, stroke, heart failure, pneumonia, uncontrolled diabetes, uremic (kidney) poisoning. A state of confusion is common following a convulsion and may come before or after unconsciousness or coma.

120

GENERAL EMERGENCY

WHAT TO DO

Call a doctor.

If possible, don't leave person alone. He might fall out of bed or from a window or start a fire by smoking in bed.

Be calm and reassuring.

Keep room brightly lit indoors to lessen his confusion and fear.

If thirsty, help him drink water or a soft drink.

DO NOT GIVE ALCOHOL OR MEDICATION IN ANY FORM.

Keep trying to explain to the person who he is, where he is, who you are and what has happened to him.

Don't try to reason him out of his strange state.

ANXIETY AND PANIC

Anxiety is the most common of all psychiatric symptoms. At worst, it produces an overwhelming sense of fear often accompanied by shakiness, sweating, palpitations and a rapid pulse. There may be a feeling of coming disaster or a sensation of not being able to breathe.

While anxiety may result from actual disease or mental confusion, its sufferers usually have no physical illness. Any emotionally difficult situation can trigger a panic attack.

"Speed" (amphetamine), LSD, or heroin can also produce panic, which sometimes leads to suicide attempts.
Sometimes marijuana or alcohol can do it.

Withdrawal from alcohol for an alcoholic is a common cause of severe anxiety.

GENERAL EMERGENCY

WHAT TO DO

Call a doctor.

If possible, see that person isn't left alone.

Be calm and reassuring.

Try to distract person with conversation until doctor comes. Most acute anxiety attacks not relating to drug abuse or alcoholism are usually over in less than an hour.

EYE PROBLEMS

Swollen or itchy lids may be due to allergy, infection or irritation.

• Apply luke-warm boric acid soaks.

• Wear dark glasses.

• See the doctor.

Most eye injuries are caused by foreign bodies. If not properly treated, you can damage your vision.

WHAT TO DO

Never rub your eye. This may force anything in it even in deeper.

• Gently hold the lashes of the upper lid and pull it over the lower lid. If object is not out after several trys then,

• Bathe the eye in luke-warm boric acid solution to float out the object.

If you can see the object, try to remove it lightly with a moistened sterilized cotton swab or the moistened corner of a clean handkerchief. If you cannot get it after two or three tries, or you can no longer see it, go to a doctor or an emergency room of a hospital.

GENERAL EMERGENCY

CHEMICAL BURNS OF THE EYE

Chemicals can cause serious damage, so speed is very important.

WHAT TO DO

Immediately wash eyes with a gentle stream of running water poured from a cup or glass or your hand. Keep this up until you're sure the chemical has been completely removed.

Close the lid and cover the injured eye with a dry, sterile gauze pad or the cleanest material you can get.

Call the doctor the second you've done this.

Until he comes, don't use oil, ointments or any other chemicals as this may make things worse.

WHEN TO CALL THE DOCTOR RIGHT AWAY

If you get a "black eye."

You have pain in the eye or over it or in the back of the head.

If you see halos around light.

If your vision suddenly blurs or gets worse.

If you have double vision.

If you see better with dark glasses or in a dimly lit room. Or do not see so well in a brightly lit room.

If you see a magenta red band on the white of the eye around the iris (the colored part). You should see doctor, but it is not an emergency.

If the whites of the eyes are red and the redness isn't caused by drinking, lack of sleep, sunburn or windburn.

If there's discharge, or sticky stuff comes from the eyes or the lids are crusted.

If a chemical or any foreign object you can't see gets into your eyes.

123

GENERAL EMERGENCY

FEVER AND CHILLS

(97 to 99 degrees F. is about normal mouth temperature.)

Fever is body temperature that goes higher than 100 degrees rectally. (Rectal temperature is one whole degree higher than mouth temperature.) Fever is an important sign of illness, and one of the ways the body fights off infection. It can come with headache, back or muscle aches, fatigue, weakness or loss of appetite. If fever rises to 104 in infants and young children (this can cause convulsions), or to 105 or above in adults, it must be brought down immediately. If chills are not followed by fever within two hours, they are probably not important.

WHAT TO DO ABOUT IT

Put patient to bed.

Take and record temperature and pulse.

Call doctor.

Until he comes, try to reduce high fever by giving aspirin. (One baby aspirin under one year of age. Two baby aspirins between the ages one and five.)Do not give aspirin if child is a known bleeder.

Give patient a sponge bath with cool water or rubbing alcohol.

Take and record temperature every half hour until repeated sponging brings fever down.

GENERAL EMERGENCY

HEART ATTACK WARNING SIGNALS

Pain from a heart attack is usually located in the front of the chest and most frequently in the center rather than one side or the other. It's usually described as a pressure or a squeezing sensation which may be associated with pains in one or both shoulders or arms and even neck. It doesn't usually have a burning quality. Nausea, vomiting, a cold sweat and difficulty in breathing may occur. Color usually turns pale.

Sharp, sticking pains or "stitches" usually don't mean heart trouble or any other serious condition. But if pain or discomfort is present continuously for twenty to thirty minutes, you should call a doctor.

- Shortness of breath, especially after light exercise.
- A pain or tightness in the chest, often extending down the left arm.
- Swelling around ankles.
- Dizziness or light-headedness.
- Double vision.
- Persistent stomach distress.
- A continual feeling of tiredness.

REMEMBER
EMERGENCY NUMBERS ON INSIDE BACK COVER

GENERAL EMERGENCY

WHAT TO DO

1. Call doctor if you feel severe or continued pain in your chest. Carefully describe your symptoms. If your doctor is not immediately available, call for an ambulance. Delay could be fatal.

2. Don't take anything by mouth until cleared to do so by your doctor. You may chew on chips of ice.

3. Get into a comfortable position in a chair or bed.

4. Avoid getting chilled. If you've been in the cold, get warm as soon as possible. If you're in a very hot place, get good ventilation or air conditioning if possible.

5. If you feel faint or dizzy, lie down — even if that means lying on the floor. However, take care not to be chilled. If you are short of breath, you'll feel better sitting up.

6. Do not walk to the doctor or bed. *Stay where you are* until the doctor or ambulance comes.

   If you have had a heart attack in the past or have been under medical care for a heart condition, get specific instructions from your doctor about what to do in case of chest pain.

FIRST AID IS NOT A SUBSTITUTE FOR MEDICAL HELP. ALWAYS SEND FOR THE DOCTOR AS QUICKLY AS POSSIBLE.

GENERAL EMERGENCY

HEMORRHOIDS (Piles)

Hemorrhoids are varicose veins of the rectum, and very common in both men and women. They may bulge out and may itch or become swollen, painful and tender. During bowel movements, hemorrhoids may be painful or may bleed without pain. When a vein in a hemorrhoid becomes clotted, the hemorrhoid becomes hard, swollen and tender to touch.

WHAT TO DO

Take "sitz" baths (sit in a bathtub filled with four or five inches of water as hot as you can stand it) from four to six times a day. This generally brings relief. If it doesn't, lie down in bed on your side and apply an ice bag to painful area.

Call your doctor.

FIRST AID IS NOT A SUBSTITUTE FOR MEDICAL HELP. ALWAYS SEND FOR THE DOCTOR AS QUICKLY AS POSSIBLE.

GENERAL EMERGENCY

HICCOUGHS

Hiccoughs are nothing more than periodic involuntary contractions of the muscle of the diaphragm. They occur in people of all ages, and even in unborn children. They rarely become serious unless they interfere with eating or sleeping or begin to cause pain.

WHAT TO DO

Hold your breath as long as you can. Three or four times.

If this doesn't work, try breathing very hard, deep and fast in between periods you hold your breath.

If that doesn't work, try swallowing a glass of ice water while holding your breath. Repeat at least once if necessary.

If there's still no relief, cover your mouth and nose with a small paper bag and breathe in and out of the bag as long as you can.

Other ways: Pull tongue way forward to gag or vomit; surprise person hiccoughing.

If nothing works, call doctor. He may give medications or an injection.

GENERAL EMERGENCY

PREGNANCY EMERGENCIES

EMERGENCY CHILDBIRTH

At some stage before the birth there will be a discharge of amniotic fluid (the breaking of the bag of waters). It averages about 1 quart so be prepared for it.

Don't worry if baby comes rapidly or without help.

If *you* are the expectant mother, get someone to stay with you until the doctor comes and have that person do the following.

WHAT TO DO:

Call doctor or ambulance.

See that mother lies down, preferably in bed.

Wash hands and keep everything as clean as possible. Slip a clean towel or sheet under mother's hips for baby to come on.

Be patient. If there's time, boil a pair of scissors and string or laces for five minutes to use later to cut the cord and tie it.

Hold baby gently as it emerges. *Don't pull on baby at any time.*

After baby comes, if it doesn't cry, hold it upside down by its feet and slap it a couple of times.

Use a clean handkerchief over your finger to wipe baby's mouth free of mucus.

If baby still isn't breathing, use gentle mouth-to-mouth breathing.

After baby cries, place it on one side of mother's abdomen face down with head slightly lowered. Cover baby to keep it warm.

Once baby is breathing regularly, wait for afterbirth to come out of mother. *Do not pull on cord.*

If you didn't have time before, boil scissors for five minutes or clean with alcohol.

129

GENERAL EMERGENCY

If doctor is on way, wait for him to tie and cut cord as there's no rush about this. *If no help is on the way,* tie a clean handkerchief strip or shoelace firmly in a square knot around the umbilical cord about four inches from the baby to stop the circulation in the cord. Do not tie or cut cord until it stops pulsing. Tie a second piece of material in a square knot around the cord six to eight inches from the baby (two to four inches beyond the first knot).

In tightening each loop of the square knot, avoid tugging on the umbilical cord. Steady one hand against the other at the knuckles as you pull the knot.

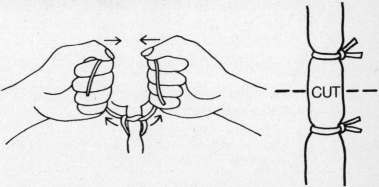

Cut the cord *between the two ties* with clean scissors.

If afterbirth is only partially out, help push it out by pressing on mother's uterus (a firm lump below the navel) with one hand. (open palm).

Once afterbirth is *all* out, gently massage mother's abdomen to help her uterus contract to minimize bleeding.

Keep mother comfortable and see that baby is warm and breathing.

Keep people away from baby and mother.

Handle baby gently and as little as possible.

There may be bleeding from a tear of mother's tissues. The pressure of a gauze pad or towel against the area will help to stop this bleeding.

130

GENERAL EMERGENCY

WHAT NOT TO DO

Don't hurry birth.

Don't interfere with birth in any way.

Don't hurry to cut cord. You can even wait until afterbirth is completely out.

Don't wash the white material off the baby. It protects baby's skin.

Do nothing to baby's eyes, ears or nose.

SYMPTOMS DURING PREGNANCY THAT MEAN TROUBLE

If any of these symptoms occur, call doctor *at once*. He'll decide whether or not they're danger signals and tell you just what to do.

Vaginal bleeding no matter how slight. (Go to bed at once and take nothing by mouth except water).

Sharp or continuous pain in abdomen.

Chills or fever.

Continuous vomiting.

Severe, continuous headache.

Dimness or blurring of vision.

Sudden escape of fluid from vagina.

GENERAL EMERGENCY

SORE THROAT

Most sore throats are not serious. However, a sore throat can be an early sign of tonsillitis, scarlet fever, trench mouth, mononucleosis, diphtheria. It can be especially dangerous for anyone who has not been immunized against diphtheria.

WHAT TO DO

Take and record temperature and pulse.

See if there's a rash on your body.

See if your throat is red or has patches of white or yellow. If this is the case, or you have a fever, call the doctor.

Report any sore throat to your doctor if you have a history of rheumatic fever or heart conditions or if sore throat lasts more than four or five days.

Do *not* take any antibiotics unless doctor tells you to.

Take aspirin or a pain reliever if there is pain. Gargle for five minutes every hour with one teaspoon of table salt to a half a glass of water *as hot as you can stand it.*

SWALLOWED OBJECTS

Any object that fits into the mouth can usually reach the stomach, go through the intestinal tract and be eliminated through the rectum. Even sharp objects such as open safety pins and pieces of glass will often pass through without much damage. However, sharp objects *may* be dangerous if swallowed.

WHAT TO DO

CATHARTICS OR LAXATIVES MUST NOT BE GIVEN UNDER ANY CIRCUMSTANCES

There is no need for emergency treatment for adults or children who have swallowed foreign objects. Just keep calm and call doctor for further advice.

132

GENERAL EMERGENCY

TOOTHACHE

EMERGENCY DENTAL TREATMENT
(Until You Can See Your Dentist)

To determine nature of toothache:

Rinse with cold water and if pain gets worse:
Rinse forcefully with lukewarm water to remove pieces of food.
Look for an open cavity in the area of the pain. Dry the area with cotton or tissue. Dip a small piece of cotton in oil of cloves and place into cavity or between teeth in area of pain.
Take two aspirin or a pain reliever if necessary.

Rinse with cold water and if pain calms down (tooth will also probably be sensitive to biting pressure):
Take two aspirin or pain reliever.
Sit up in easy chair or prop yourself up high in bed. (Lying down increases pain.)
Rinse with ice water or suck on crushed ice.
If gum or face are swollen, apply a heating pad or hot water bottle to side of face.

What to do for loss of filling or broken tooth:

If there is no pain but only jagged edges, chew a piece of candlewax, beeswax, or paraffin along with some strands of sterile absorbent cotton.
Use this material to cover jagged edges that may irritate tongue or cheek and to prevent entrance of food.

TAKE CARE OF TEETH

There's no foolproof way to prevent cavities. Visit your dentist every six months. Brush your teeth, whenever possible, after eating. If unable to brush, swish warm water in and out between your teeth to get rid of bits of food. Brush teeth away from gums. Bottom up; top down. Don't eat lots of starches, candy, cake, soda.

GENERAL EMERGENCY

What to do for pain from pulled tooth or mouth injury:

Take two aspirins or other pain reliever.
If bleeding, make a ball of sterile gauze to place over the open area (where tooth was) and bite together forcefully for a half hour till clot forms. Repeat if necessary. Do not rinse mouth as this will loosen blood clot. If clot does not form, call your dentist.
Apply an ice pack fifteen minutes on and fifteen minutes off to side of face if there is pain.

What to do in case of loose porcelain jacket, crown, or fixed bridge:

Do not use any commercial cements (they may injure tooth or ruin crown).
Clean inside of crown and try denture adhesive paste to hold jacket in position for appearance. (Remove crown or bridge when you eat as you may swallow it).
Get to dentist to have it recemented.

VOMITING, NAUSEA, STOMACH PAINS

These symptoms can happen separately or all together in cases of "simple upset," intestinal flu, food poisoning, irritable colon, female disorders, stomach ulcers, gall bladder trouble or appendicitis. Correct diagnosis takes all the skill of a fine doctor, so don't try to guess on your own. If nausea, pain in the stomach or abdomen or vomiting continues, recurs, or puzzles you, call your doctor.

• *Don't take or give a laxative or cathartic unless your doctor tells you to.*

• Don't take or give anything by mouth (food, water, alcohol, liquids, medicine) unless your doctor tells you to.

• Take and write down your temperature and pulse. This can help your doctor know what to do.

• Lie down or get into bed.

134

FAMILY HEALTH SUPPLEMENT

HOW TO CHOOSE A FAMILY DOCTOR

Don't wait for an emergency before you find a doctor. It's important to have a family doctor because he keeps records and can notice any changes in normal health patterns. If you move, be sure your new doctor sends for your family medical history. It is always wise to ask your present doctor if he can recommend someone in the area you move to. You can check on any doctor's background at the library in the American Medical Directory.

Feel free to discuss his fees, whether or not he will make house calls, what hospital he is associated with, if he has doctors covering for him when he's away. Finally, decide whether you like the doctor you interview. Any doctor should welcome an intelligent interest.

FINDING A DOCTOR IN AN EMERGENCY

Call your local hospital, medical school, or county or state medical society. Or look up a doctor under "Physicians" in your telephone directory.

In a big city it is often faster to call an ambulance and go to the emergency department of your hospital.

CHECK-UPS FOR A LONGER, HAPPIER LIFE

If you've changed doctors for any reason, it's a good idea to have a complete medical examination. Your new doctor will then know something about you in case of an emergency and you will learn something about him. One out of every four people have some kind of chronic disease. Your chances of staying out of this 25% group are much better if you have yourself checked by a doctor regularly.

135

FAMILY HEALTH SUPPLEMENT

CHECK-UPS FOR INFANTS AND CHILDREN:

Age	Frequency
First year or 6 months	every 4 to 6 weeks, then every 3 months
Second year	every 3 months
3 to 6 years	every 6 to 12 months
7 to 18 years	once a year

CHECK-UPS FOR ADULTS:

Age	Frequency
18-35 years	every 2 or 3 years
35-50 years	every year
50 and over	once or twice a year on the advice of your doctor

CANCER WARNING SIGNALS

100,000 Americans die of cancer NEEDLESSLY every year. Mostly because it wasn't discovered and treated soon enough. (Sometimes a call to your doctor can reassure you that certain symptoms are *not* due to cancer.) Get a complete check-up once a year.

- Any sore that doesn't heal.
- Any lump or thickening in the breast or elsewhere.
- Bloody discharge from any body opening.
- Change in the color or size of a wart or mole.
- Persistent indigestion or difficulty in swallowing.
- Persistent coughing or hoarseness.
- Change in normal bowel movements or habits.

FAMILY HEALTH SUPPLEMENT

IMMUNIZATION

Once a child comes down with measles, he will probably never have them again. This is because the body, during an illness, builds up a defense system against the disease with something called antibodies. This is immunization. One does not have to wait to get a disease in order to gain immunity. Scientists discovered that antigens can teach the body to produce the desired antibodies if disease attacks. At birth, a mother gives her child an immunity to the diseases she has had. This is called passive or temporary immunity and lasts about six months. Before protection fades, a doctor reinforces the child's defenses with a series of immunization injections. Protection is continually kept up with "booster" shots, given at different times through a person's lifetime. Immunization is very important for adults as well as children. Half the deaths from tetanus (lockjaw) every year happen to adults who have never been immunized or have neglected "booster" shots. Particularly important shots for adults: mumps (for adolescents, particularly males), tetanus, diphtheria, smallpox. Other shots are sometimes necessary for traveling to other countries. Other major disease protection is listed in charts below.

IMMUNIZATION SCHEDULE

ADULTS

Diphtheria-tetanus every 10 years
Smallpox booster every 3 to 10 years
Rubella—only in women who have not had German measles and who are not pregnant and will not be for 3 months
Mumps——in men who have not had it
Typhoid-paratyphoid fever——for foreign travel
Influenza——each fall for persons subject to risk or with debilitating or chronic diseases

137

FAMILY HEALTH SUPPLEMENT

Be sure to see your doctor at the right times so you are protected against these diseases.

IMMUNIZATION NECESSARY FOR INFANTS AND CHILDREN

2 MONTHS	Diphtheria-tetanus-whooping cough Oral poliomyelitis
3 MONTHS	Diphtheria-tetanus-whooping cough
4 MONTHS	Diphtheria-tetanus-whooping cough Oral poliomyelitis
6 MONTHS	Oral poliomyelitis
12 MONTHS	Live measles vaccine Tuberculin test
15-18 MONTHS	Diphtheria-tetanus-whooping cough Oral poliomyelitis Smallpox
4-6 YEARS	Diphtheria-tetanus-whooping cough Oral poliomyelitis Smallpox
5-9 YEARS	Rubella (German measles)
12 YEARS	Diphtheria-tetanus Smallpox Mumps (Some pediatricians now give mumps vaccine anytime from age 1 to 12)

138

FAMILY HEALTH SUPPLEMENT

DRUGS

DRUG	SLANG NAME	DANGERS
COCAINE (This is the oldest local anesthetic.)	Coke Snow The leaf	Dizziness and mental confusion. Large doses often cause severe depression and nervous exhaustion which can last for several days. Overdose can cause convulsions, *even death* due to paralysis of respiratory center. Psychologically but not physically addicting.
AMPHETA-MINES (Used to control weight, fight fatigue, reduce some types of depression)	Speed Bennies Pep pills Dexies Hearts Co-Pilots Lid Poppers	Stimulants can drive users to do things beyond physical limits. Heavy doses can cause temporary mental illness. Withdrawal from drug can result in suicidal depression. High doses can cause death. Psychologically but not physically addicting, although users must use increasingly larger doses for effect.

Drug Emergencies, see page 117.

FAMILY HEALTH SUPPLEMENT

EFFECT ON BODY

Cocaine is an "up." Causes quickened pulse, accelerated circulation, sharpened reactions, dilated pupils, increased activity, restlessness, panting, shakes.

EFFECT ON NERVOUS SYSTEM

Over-confidence in mental and physical capacities. Feeling of well being, loss of sense of time. Depression. Large doses produce hallucinations and feelings of persecution.

Amphetamines are "ups" that increase heart rate, blood pressure, throbbing of heart, enlarge pupils, dry mouth, cause sweating, headaches, paleness, diarrhea, increased activity, restlessness, shaky hands, unclear speech.

Feeling of alertness, self-confidence, sometimes followed by depression, unreal idea of one's strength and mental ability. Heavy dose can cause person to fear and see imaginary things.

DRUGS CONTINUED OVER

FAMILY HEALTH SUPPLEMENT

DRUGS (Continued)

DRUG	SLANG NAME	DANGERS
OPIATES Codeine is used to reduce pain and suppress cough; Morphine is a pain-killer; Heroin has *no* medical use in U.S.A.	Schoolboy M Horse H Stuff Junk Harry Joy Powder	*Death can result from overdoses.* Hepatitis from injections with unsterilized needles. Judgment, self-control and attention span worsen. Often malnutrition. Users become physically dependent. Body needs drug just to feel comfort. Psychological need develops and body builds a tolerance so that more drugs are needed. Cure rate very low.
BARBITU-RATES Pentobarbital Secobarbital Ambarbital	Barbs Goof Balls Blues Yellow Jackets Phennies Candy Blue Heavens	*Overdoses can cause death.* Barbiturates are the leading cause of accidental poisoning and suicide in the U.S. Reality is "mixed-up," and user can lose count of pills taken and easily take an overdose. Barbiturates can lead to physical as well as psychological dependence. Body needs increasingly higher doses. Some experts feel this dependency is the most difficult to cure.

Drug Emergencies, see page 117.

141

FAMILY HEALTH SUPPLEMENT

EFFECT ON BODY

Opiates are "downs" and decrease hunger, thirst, sex drive and feeling of pain. User often goes into stupor or sleep.

EFFECT ON NERVOUS SYSTEM

User experiences a high, dreamy state. He is generally passive and lazy, but becomes extremely aggressive and will go to any length to get drugs when he needs them.

Barbiturates are "downs." They cause depressed action of skeletal and heart muscles, slowed heart rate and breathing, lower blood pressure, slurred speech, staggering, deep sleep.

Depressed action of nerves; confusion; ability to think, work, and concentrate is lessened. Emotional control is weakened. Responses are slowed down.

DRUGS CONTINUED OVER

FAMILY HEALTH SUPPLEMENT

DRUGS (Continued)

DRUG	SLANG NAME	DANGERS
LYSERGIC ACID DIETHYLA-MIDE Hallucinogens have no proven medical use, but are still being tested. (Other hallucinogens: DMT, STP, DOM, Mescaline, Psilocybin, Hashish)	LSD Acid Cubes Big D Sugar	Hallucinogens are not habit forming physically, but can lead to deep psychological dependence. They can lead to panic, paranoia, "flash-backs," death. Users sometimes have delusions that nothing can harm them and take chances.
MARIJUANA This is a "mild" hallucinogen.	Pot Grass Weed Mary Jane Tea Reefers	Marijuana is not physically addictive, but psychological need can develop (milder than LSD and other "strong" hallucinogens). Research on long-term effects being done.

Drug Emergencies, see page 117.

143

FAMILY HEALTH SUPPLEMENT

EFFECT ON BODY

Mind benders cause changes in perception and consciousness. Pulse, heart beat, blood pressure and temperature increase. Pupils dilate. Hands and feet shake, face gets flushed or pale, also cold, sweaty palms, shivering, wet mouth, irregular breathing, nausea.

EFFECT ON NERVOUS SYSTEM

Increase and distortion of senses. Loss of ability to see fact from fantasy. Loss of sense of time. Often feel two opposing emotions at the same time. Inability to reason logically. Everything is either good or bad.

This mild mind bender causes rapid heart beat, lowering of body temperature, reddening of eyes, changed blood sugar level, stimulated appetite, dehydrated body, drowsiness, lack of coordination, inflammation of mucous membranes and bronchial tubes.

State of intoxication, feeling of well-being, hilarity, confusion, distortion of time and space, loss of judgment, memory. Sometimes severe depression, moodiness, fear of death, panic. Sometimes there is no mood change.

144

BASIC FIRST AID SUPPLIES

BASIC FIRST AID SUPPLIES

FIRST AID EMERGENCY BOX:

First aid supplies should be kept in a box that is kept in a special place — *apart from* other medicines and supplies. The box should be large enough so that everything can be seen clearly and found quickly.

FIRST AID EMERGENCY BOX CONTENTS:

1. Sterile gauze pads in different sizes — from 2" x 2" up to 24" x 72" (can be bought packaged at drugstore).
2. Scissors.
3. Tweezers.
4. Safety pins.
5. Thermometer.
6. Petroleum jelly.
7. Salt tablets.
8. Syrup of Ipecac.
9. Roll of adhesive tape.
10. Adhesive compresses–different sizes.
11. Box of adhesive bandages — different sizes.
12. Roll of sterile absorbent cotton.
13. Triangular bandages.
14. Aromatic spirits of ammonia.
15. Roll of gauze bandages — 1" wide.
16. Oil of cloves or toothache drops or toothache gel (may be bought at drugstore).

17. Three-inch elastic bandage.
18. Soap.
19. Baking soda.
20. Alcohol pads.
21. Calamine lotion.
22. Inflatable splints

Take a First Aid Emergency Box and a copy of this book when you go on a car or camping trip. Check your home and travel Emergency Box frequently and replace opened or used items.

145

EMERGENCY

EMERGENCY NUMBERS:

Dial 0 for operator if you can't reach help. Tell her it's an emergency. Be *sure* she has right address. If you're alone and can't stay on the phone, leave it off the hook *after* giving operator information.

**FAMILY
DOCTOR**_____**Phone**_____

   Address_____

DOCTOR_____**Phone**_____

   Address_____

DOCTOR_____**Phone**_____

   Address_____

AMBULANCE_____**Phone**_____

HOSPITAL_____**Phone**_____

   Address_____

POLICE_____**Phone**_____

_____

FIRE DEPT._____**Phone**_____

_____